CARDIOLOGY RESEARCH AND CLINICAL DEVELOPMENTS SERIES

CARDIAC REHABILITATION

CARDIOLOGY RESEARCH AND CLINICAL DEVELOPMENTS SERIES

Focus on Atherosclerosis Research
Leon V. Clark (Editor)
2004. ISBN: 1-59454-044-6

Cholesterol in Atherosclerosis and Coronary Heart Disease
Jean P. Kovala (Editor)
2005. ISBN: 1-59454-302-X

Frontiers in Atherosclerosis Research
Karin F. Kepper (Editor)
2007. ISBN: 1-60021-371-5

Cardiac Arrhythmia Research Advances
Lynn A. Vespry (Editor)
2007. ISBN: 1-60021-794-X

Cardiac Arrhythmia Research Advances
Lynn A. Vespry (Editor)
2007. ISBN: 978-1-60692-539-3
(Online Book)

Heart Disease in Women
Benjamin V. Lardner and Harrison R. Pennelton (Editors)
2009. ISBN: 978-1-60692-066-4

Heart Disease in Women
Benjamin V. Lardner and Harrison R. Pennelton (Editors)
2010. ISBN: 978-1-60741-090-4
(Online Book)

Cardiomyopathies: Causes, Effects and Treatment
Peter H. Bruno and Matthew T. Giordano (Editors)
2009. ISBN: 978-1-60692-193-7

Cardiomyopathies: Causes, Effects and Treatment
Peter H. Bruno and Matthew T. Giordano (Editors)
2009. ISBN: 978-1-60876-433-4
(Online Book)

Transcatheter Coil Embolization of Visceral Arterial Aneurysms
Shigeo Takebayashi, Izumi Torimoto and Kiyotaka Imoto (Editors)
2009. ISBN: 978-1-60741-439-1

Transcatheter Coil Embolization of Visceral Arterial Aneurysms
Shigeo Takebayashi, Izumi Torimoto and Kiyotaka Imoto (Editors)
2009. ISBN: 978-1-978-1-60876-797-7
(Online Book)

Heart Disease in Men
Alice B. Todd and Margo H. Mosley (Editors)
2009. ISBN: 978-1-60692-297-2

Angina Pectoris: Etiology, Pathogenesis and Treatment
Alice P. Gallos and Margaret L. Jones (Editors)
2009. ISBN: 978-1-60456-674-1

Coronary Artery Bypasses
Russell T. Hammond and James B Alton (Editors)
2009. ISBN: 978-1-60741-064-5

Congenital Heart Defects: Etiology, Diagnosis and Treatment
Hiroto Nakamura (Editor)
2009. ISBN: 978-1-60692-559-1

Congenital Heart Defects: Etiology, Diagnosis and Treatment
Hiroto Nakamura (Editor)
2009. ISBN: 978-1-60876-434-1
(Online Book))

Atherosclerosis: Understanding Pathogenesis and Challenge for Treatment
Slavica Mitrovska, Silvana Jovanova Inge Matthiesen and Christian Libermans
2009. ISBN: 978-1-60692-677-2

Practical Rapid ECG Interpretation (PREI)
Abraham G. Kocheril and Ali A. Sovari
2009. ISBN: 978-1-60741-021-8

Heart Transplantation: Indications and Contraindications, Procedures and Complications
Catherine T. Fleming (Editor)
2009. ISBN 978-1-60741-228-1

Heart Transplantation: Indications and Contraindications, Procedures and Complications
Catherine T. Fleming (Editor)
2010. ISBN 978-1-60876-591-1
(Online Book)

Heart Disease in Children
Marius D. Oliveira and William S. Copley (Editors)
2009. ISBN: 978-1-60741-504-6

Heart Disease in Children
Marius D. Oliveira and William S. Copley (Editors)
2009. ISBN: 978-1-61668-225-5
(Online Book)

Handbook of Cardiovascular Research
Jorgen Brataas and Viggo Nanstveit (Editors)
2009. ISBN: 978-1-60741-792-7

Comprehensive Models of Cardiovascular and Respiratory Systems: Their Mechanical Support and Interactions
Marek Darowsk
and Gianfranco Ferrari (Editors)
2009. ISBN: 978-1-60876-212-5

Cardiovascular Signals in Diabetes Mellitus: A New Tool to Detect Autonomic Neuropathy
Michal Javorka, Ingrid Tonhajzerova,
Zuzana Turianikova, Kamil Javorka,
Natasa Honzikova
and Mathias Baumert
2010. ISBN: 978-1-60876-788-5

Cardiac Rehabilitation
Jonathon T. Halliday (Editor)
2010. ISBN: 978-1-60741-918-1

CARDIOLOGY RESEARCH AND CLINICAL DEVELOPMENTS SERIES

CARDIAC REHABILITATION

JONATHON T. HALLIDAY
EDITOR

Nova Science Publishers, Inc.
New York

Library of Congress Cataloging-in-Publication Data

Available upon request.

ISBN: 978-1-60741-918-1

Published by Nova Science Publishers, Inc. ✝ New York

Contents

Preface

Cardiac rehabilitation (CR)is a branch of rehabilitation medicine dealing with optimizing physical function in patients with cardiac diseases. CR services are generally provided in an outpatient setting as comprehensive, long-term programs involving medical evaluation, prescribed exercise, cardiac risk factor modification, education and counseling. While the "glue" of cardiac rehabilitation is exercise, programs are evolving to become comprehensive prevention centers where all aspects of preventive cardiology care are delivered. This includes nutritional therapies, weight loss programs, management of lipid abnormalities with diet and medication, blood pressure control, diabetes management and stress management. Patients typically enter cardiac rehabilitation in the weeks following an acute coronary event such as an myocardial infarction (heart attack), coronary bypass surgery, coronary stent placement or replacement of a heart valve. This new and important book gathers the latest research from around the globe in the study of cardiac rehabilitation and highlights such topics as: cardiac rehabilitation in women, deep vein thrombosis after cardiac surgery, cardiac rehabilitation in children with congenital heart disease and others.

Chapter I - One of the consequences of disturbances on the neurocardiogenic tonus is orthostatic dysregulation Blood Pressure (BP). Postural BP dysregulation is defined by a persistent (≥ 3 minutes) change in BP which is greater than 20 mmHg for its systolic component or ≥ 10 mmHg for its diastolic compound. The most common well-known subtype of orthostatic BP dysregulation is postural hypotension (P.Hypo), but Postural BP hypertension (P.Hype) is also increasingly being recognized to be crossectionally associated with adverse outcomes. Several studies have shown an association between cognitive impairment and dementia, on one side, and dysregulation in postural BP, on another side. Sudden and relatively prolonged (more than 3 minutes) changes in brain perfusion caused by P.Hypo may contribute to cause small, asymptomatic, lacunar strokes or even contribute to leukoaraiosis/White Matter Hyperintensities (WMH) on MRI. It is less clear if disruptions in cerebral blood flow caused by P.Hype can also contribute to a brain's small-vessel disease. For instance, microhemorrhages, especially if amyloid angiopathy co-occurs, may be precipitated by such sudden, overactive increases in orthostatic BP and, consequently, in the pressure of brain perfusion. Conversely, many neurodegenerative diseases may course with dysautonomia, including postural BP dysregulation. Lewy body disease (LBD) is the second most common neurodegenerative dementia (~ 20% of all dementia) and significant Lewy-body pathology co-occurs in approximately half of the cases diagnosed with Alzheimer's disease (AD) in post-mortem studies. Evidence is accumulating that AD, in its earliest stages, involves the brainstem. Since the neurovascular BP regulator control is located at the medulla oblongata, it is not surprising that many patients diagnosed with early-stage AD already have dysregulation in orthostatic BP control. Patients with Vascular Dementia (VD), which, together with LBD is the second most common dementing subtype, seem to have important impairment in the regulation of cerebral blood flow, especially if they also have unilateral or bilateral carotid stenosis greater than 50–70%. In patients with bilateral carotid stenosis greater than 70%, routine seated BP levels are inversely associated with ischemic strokes. Therefore, as exposed above, several lines of evidence point toward a vicious circle relationship between postural BP dysregulation and cognitive impairment/dementia. Since heart failure can contribute to P.Hypo, interventions that, in the long run, increase both the cardiac output and the neurocardiovascular tonus, such as aerobic exercise, may ameliorate P.Hypo. Moreover, dysregulation on the neurocardiovascular tonus, like that existent in overactive P.Hype, may also respond favorably to interventions that aim to improve both the cardiac function and the neurocardiovascular tonus, such as aerobic exercise.

Chapter II - Cardiovascular diseases (CVD) become the leading cause of death in the worldwide over the last decades. CVD in women brings about more disadvantages compare to men; such as later onset age, existence of other diseases and co-morbid conditions accompanying to older age. Symptoms of CVD display itself differently in women than in men, misdiagnosis is common in women. Cardiac rehabilitation (CR), targets to optimize the physical, psychological, social functioning of patients and to reduce cardiovascular morbidity and mortality. Women have a significantly lower rate of referral, are less likely to enroll and drop out before completing CR programs compared with their male counterparts.

This review enlightened CVD rates in women, different aspects of women's CVD, cardiac rehabilitation objectives, components, benefits, barriers and recommendations among women.

It is well known that, risk factors play role in the development and progression of CVD. Primary and secondary prevention categories of the CR are based on the development or manifestation of atherosclerotic CVD. Both prevention efforts have same strategies. They involve cardiovascular risk reduction, encourage healthy behavior and conformity with those behaviors and support an active life style in patients with high-risk profile or CVD. Female coronary patients have higher risk factors than male. At menopause, parallel to the changes in body composition, lipid measures, insulin resistance and decline in physical activity, risk factors become more serious. CR programs lessen the risks, improve exercise tolerance, reduce stress, and increase quality of life levels. Literature supports that women benefit from CR as much as men do. Realization of health benefits is dependent on attendance and compliance to basic components of CR program (exercise training, diet etc). Some barriers included noncardiac morbidity, less social support, advanced age, high prevalence of depression and family responsibilities lessen the adherence rates in women. When this gender difference in participation rates were considered, primary prevention of CVD is crucial. 2007 The American Heart Association (AHA) guideline for CVD prevention in women, recommended the determination of women's CVD risk levels as high, intermediate, lower and optimal risk. This report also advised to take measures against CVD in either women at high risk or apparently healthy women. Lifestyle interventions in new guideline comprised smoking, physical activity, rehabilitation, dietary intake, weight reduction, omega-3 fatty acids and depression. Consequently, there is a need for future research focus on not only primary/secondary prevention but also increase the compliance of women with CR programs.

Chapter III - It is increasingly clear that exercise capacity is impaired not only in systolic, but also in diastolic heart failure (DHF). In DHF, the inability of heart to increase output during exercise is primarily due to the limited Left Ventricular (LV) end-diastolic volume, despite a normal LV contractility and increased filling pressure. Healthy subjects performing exercise activity usually present an increase in heart rate that shortens diastolic filling, which results in an augmented LV filling rate that maintains or even increases LV stroke volume; this is accomplished by an enhancement of LV relaxation and a decrease in early-diastolic pressure. The mechanisms underlying an enhanced LV relaxation during exercise could involve both sympathetic stimulation and increased elastic recoil due to contractions to a lower volume. However, the adaptations in LV relaxation and early-diastolic pressure described above are not found when DHF patients are put on exercise. Indeed, LV relaxation may be acutely worsened and early-diastolic LV pressure may even increase in such a situation. Diastolic dysfunction is usually a consequence of aging, hypertrophy, ischemia, or a combination of them, and studies have shown that well-planed, long-term, increasing exercise training could favorably influence all of these effects. Accordingly, several studies have evaluated diastolic function in endurance-trained and power-trained (static exercise) patients. Among other mechanisms, endurance training prolongs the time for diastolic filling by inducing a relative sinus bradycardia secondary to either increased vagal tone or volume-induced baroceptor activation. In contrast, static exercise training results in an increased LV wall thickness relative to radius, similar to the changes following pressure-overload hypertrophy, but despite an increase in LV mass, none of the studies have demonstrated abnormal diastolic function after static training. However, repetitive lifting of greater than a few pounds should be avoided in DHF patients due to potential deleterious effects of isometric exercise on LV size and function. Therefore, based upon available data, aerobic, dynamic cardiac rehabilitation should be offered to patients with stable class II to III DHF who do not have advanced arrhythmias or another limitation to exercise. Clinical trials with appropriate outcome end-points, such as increased longevity, decreased symptoms, or improved QOL, are welcome in order to definitively prove the benefits of exercise training in patients with isolated DHF.

Chapter IV - There is already a large body of evidence suggesting that hypertension among the youngest-old (65–80 years-old) should be treated no differently from that of younger adults. This includes the current definition of hypertension (≥ 140 mmHg for systolic or ≥ 90 mmHg for diastolic Blood Pressure [BP]) also for this age group. Even though orientations from the 'VII Joint on Hypertension' have recommended the extrapolation of this evidence also for the oldest-old group (≥ 80 y.o), until recently there was no definite evidence that treating hypertension in this age group would reduce overall mortality. In fact, a meta-analysis of several mega clinical trials, which have included small subgroups of very elderly people, has found a reverse relationship between treating hypertension and overall mortality. Very recently, the HyVET study has found that treating otherwise healthy very elderly hypertensive (systolic BP 160–210 mmHg as inclusion criteria) people at a goal of 150 x 80 mmHg of systolic and diastolic BP, respectively, reduces overall mortality over an average 1.8 year period. However, several considerations should arise when interpreting data from this study. First, this study included vastly healthy elderly people, having excluded subjects with heart failure (HF), dementia, and frail, institutionalized, elderly people. HF and dementia are possibly the two main confounders of the relationship between BP and mortality among the very elderly. BP tends to decrease in dilated hypertensive myocardiopathy, as it does in malnutrition states associated with advanced dementia. In fact, a study has found that, in the general very elderly population, hypertension was only associated with increased overall mortality after excluding people who have deceased within a 3-year period from baseline, a disproportional part of them apparently from HF and dementia. Aging is a heterogeneous process, and considering only chronological age may not be adequate in analyzing the relationship between BP and mortality in the very elderly. For instance, the relationship between BP and risk of ischemic stroke is the inverse among people with bilateral carotid stenosis ≥ 70%, regardless of age. As a general rule, it may be reasonable deciding to treat otherwise healthy very elderly hypertensive people (without HF, significant carotid stenosis, or moderate-to-advanced dementia) with at least 2 consecutive systolic BP measures ≥ 160 mmHg. In this specific age group, the therapeutic goal should be 150 x 80 mmHg, as evidenced by the HyVET study. Lower BP levels might be associated with an increased risk of hypoperfusional stroke even among otherwise healthy very elderly people, since cerebral blood flow autoregulation is lost in the presence of significant cerebrovascular disease — a finding not uncommon in this age group.

Chapter VI - Metabolic Syndrome (Met.S) consists of a cluster of symptoms including abdominal obesity, glucose intolerance, low HDL-cholesterol, high triglycerides, and high blood pressure. All of these components seem to be caused, at least partially, by the same pathophysiologic process, named Insulin Resistance (IR). IR has been recognized as having a central role in regulating biological aging. Hyperglycemia and hyperinsulinism are two consequences of IR, both of which being associated with an increased formation of Reactive Oxygen Species (ROS) and Advance Glucose Endproducts (AGEs). ROS and AGE are the key points for each of the two main theories of aging: oxidative stress and protein glycation, respectively. IR is, in fact, a mechanism intrinsically associated with calorie ingestion; calorie restriction being the only proved way to extend life in mammals, including primates. Diabetic cardiomyopathy is well-known to be associated with myocardial aging and Diastolic Heart Failure (DHF). Evidences are accumulating that milder forms of IR and hyperglycemia are also associated with increased myocardial cell oxidative stress and protein glycation. Hyperinsulinism also causes capillary endothelial proliferation, contributing to microvascular ischemic myocardiopathy and, consequently, diastolic dysfunction.

Hypertension, another component of Met.S, is the most common cause of (concentric) hypertrophic myocardiopathy, which can further impair ventricular complacence, contributing to DHF. Managing Met.S components in an integrated approach may contribute to cardiac rehabilitation in many ways. Losing weight by itself can ameliorate DHF by both direct and indirect mechanisms. Weight reduction would decrease the need for a continuously elevated cardiac output at rest which, by itself, would improve symptoms in heart failure. Adequately managing Met.S components may improve diastolic relaxation through two main mechanisms. First, tight control of blood pressure would prevent myocardial remodeling and even regress, to some degree, this process, improving diastolic function. Second, strict long-term glycemic control has the potential to decelerate myocardial aging and, additionally, improve diastolic function both by regressing cardiac microangiopathy and intracellular glucose utilization by the myocardial cell. Exercise is an essential part in the cardiac rehabilitation plan of the patient with IR-associated myocardiopathy. Independent of weight reduction, dynamic exercise is able to improve IR, diastolic function, and peripheral energy utilization, all mechanisms collaborating to rehabilitation on DHF.

Chapter VII – Introduction: Venous thromboembolism (VTE) is an important cause of morbidity and mortality after many general surgical procedures and can be a complication of central venous catheterization(CVC) .

In cardiac surgery the CVC is frequently placed in the right internal jugular vein, but procedure has still not been properly assessed as regards either the risk of deep vein thrombosis catheter- related (DVT–CVC related) and Pulmonary embolism (PE).We assessed the impact of right internal jugular vein CVC-related DVT and the risk of PE in patients after coronary artery bypass grafts (CABG), valve replacement surgery, or both; we also assessed therapeutic options.

Material and Methods: We considered 1000 patients after cardiac surgery and admitted to intensive cardiac rehabilitation 5 to 7 days later (mean 5.8);960 were enrolled.

All had CVC in right internal jugular vein: a triple-lumen central venous catheter 14 gauge was inserted immediately before surgery and removed 3 to 4 days later;within 3 days after admission the patients were checked by ultrasonography (US) exploring neck vessels.

DVT diagnosed was classified as at low risk of embolism when it was only a small strip less than 2 cm long (limited) or at high risk of embolism when it was free-floating or sub-occlusive the lumen. PE had been confirmed by pulmonary angio-CT scan.

Results: 461 patients (48%) had asymptomatic CVC-related DVT. None of the patients with CVC-related DVT and anticoagulant therapy presented clinical signs or symptoms of PE while in rehabilitation, or after three months. Among the patients with CVC-related DVT receiving antiplatelet and considered at low risk ,PE was seen in the six cases; among all those considered at high risk of embolism , the antiplatelet was replaced with low-molecular-weight fractionated heparin and warfarin (INR 2,5-3,5), continued for at least three months or until there were no longer any US signs of thrombosis. This group had no cases of clinically manifest PE either while in hospital or at three months.

Discussion: Very little is known about the prevalence of thrombotic events in CVC-related DVT of the neck after cardiac surgery. In the present study with several types of heart surgery, 48% had DVT related to a CVC in the right internal jugular vein; this is significantly higher than the figure for lower-extremity DVT in the same type of population . About 1,200,000 heart operations are performed every year in the U.S.A.; therefore, we can assume that more than 500,000 heart operations each year may be complicated with CVC-related DVT.

The causes or factors responsible for this complication are still not clear, just as the real reason why the thrombus forms is not known. Controversy also surrounds the question of how best to prevent CVC-related DVT:the utility for preventing CVC-related DVT with unfractionated heparin and warfarin remains to be established .Our findings suggest that neither heparin given during surgery nor anticoagulant therapy with heparin and warfarin immediately after surgery are very reliable for preventing venous thrombosis; early antiplatelet therapy also had no significant preventive effect. Anticoagulation with warfarin does seem to prevent clinically manifest PE in all patients with CVC-related DVT, regardless of type of thrombus or heart surgery. In addition, sonographic screening of the CVC removal in intensive cardiac unit may be useful for avoiding PE after CVC-related DVT.

Chapter IX – Objective: The aim of this study was to estimate the prevalence of depression and anxiety among patients in cardiac rehabilitation at Reykjalundur Rehabilitation Center and to study the impact of a 4-5 weeks inpatient cardiac rehabilitation program on these symptoms. Secondly we wished to compare the concordance of our clinical diagnosis with the results of a standardized psychometric scale, Hospital Anxiety and Depression scale, HAD.

Materials and Methods: Of 224 patients in one year, 200 (89.3%) were included in the study, 151 men and 49 women. The patients were first evaluated by a doctor and a nurse separately at the arrival and a clinical evaluation was made jointly. Shortly after arrival and before departure a HAD questionnaire was to be answered. All new psychiatric treatment was recorded.

Results: Prevalence of depression as measured by HAD was reduced from 9.5% to 3.1% and anxiety from 11.6% to 2.5%. The sensitivity of clinical diagnosis of depression as compared to the results of HAD was 73.7% and specificity 87.3%. For anxiety the sensitivity was 86.4% and specificity was 79.2%. The predictive value of a positive clinical diagnosis of depressions was 37.8% and anxiety 33.9%, but predictive value of a negative clinical diagnosis was 96.9% and anxiety 97.9% respectively.

Conclusion: The prevalence of depression and anxiety is similar or somewhat lower than in other studies on patients with cardiac diseases. The agreement of clinical diagnosis and HAD questionnaire was acceptable and the questionnaire will not be used routinely. A comprehensive cardiac rehabilitation program seems to substantially reduce symptoms of depression and anxiety among patients in cardiac rehabilitation at Reykjalundur.

Chapter X - As the majority of the patients with congenital heart disease belong to the paediatric age group, exercise testing equipment and exercise protocols have to be adapted for children.

Functional performance should be assessed by performing exercise testing with measurement of gas exchange. Nowadays, new concepts for exercise testing in the paediatric age group are analysis of gas exchange during the non-steady state of exercise and determination of the kinetics of gas exchange during the recovery phase of exercise.

In some groups of patients with congenital heart disease, suboptimal values have been found for aerobic exercise capacity, which can be ascribed to hemodynamic dysfunction or residual hemodynamic lesions after surgery (e.g. in transposition of the great arteries, tetralogy of Fallot, and Fontan repair for univentricular heart). In other types of pathologies medically imposed restriction of intensive physical exercise or competitive sports may determine to some extent a subnormal value of exercise performance.

Finally in some other types of congenital heart disease without overt hemodynamic dysfunction (e.g. ventricular septal defect or atrial septal defect, with normal pressures in the pulmonary circulation) a suboptimal value for aerobic capacity is often related to overprotection of the parents or environment of the child. Therefore, except for some cases with medically imposed restriction of intensive physical exercise, most patients are encouraged to be fully active during leisure time and to participate in all types of physical exercise at school.

Exercise intensity is usually defined as the highest level of physical activity at which the child is still able to talk during physical activity.

Formal rehabilitation programs are generally indicated after surgical correction of the defect during the hospitalisation period.

In: Cardiac Rehabilitaiton
Editor: J. T. Halliday, pp. 1-38
ISBN: 978-1-60741-918-1

Chapter I

Postural Blood Pressure Dysregulation and Dementia: Evidence for a Vicious Circle, and Implications for Neurocardiovascular Rehabilitation

***Jarbas S. Roriz-Filho*[1], *Silvio R. Bernardes-Silva-Filho*[1], *Idiane Rosset*[2] *and Matheus Roriz-Cruz*[2*]**

[1]Division of Geriatrics. Department of Internal Medicine. School of Medicine of Ribeirão Preto at University of São Paulo-RP, Brazil
[2]Division of Gerontological Nursing. Faculty of Nursing. Brazilian Federal University of Rio Grande do Sul State, Brazil

One of the consequences of disturbances on the neurocardiogenic tonus is orthostatic dysregulation Blood Pressure (BP). Postural BP dysregulation is defined by a persistent (≥ 3 minutes) change in BP which is greater than 20 mmHg for its systolic component or ≥ 10 mmHg for its diastolic compound. The most common well-known subtype of

* Corresponding author: Division of Gerontological Nursing. Faculty of Nursing. Brazilian Federal University of Rio Grande do Sul State, Brazil

orthostatic BP dysregulation is postural hypotension (P.Hypo), but Postural BP hypertension (P.Hype) is also increasingly being recognized to be crossectionally associated with adverse outcomes. Several studies have shown an association between cognitive impairment and dementia, on one side, and dysregulation in postural BP, on another side. Sudden and relatively prolonged (more than 3 minutes) changes in brain perfusion caused by P.Hypo may contribute to cause small, asymptomatic, lacunar strokes or even contribute to leukoaraiosis/White Matter Hyperintensities (WMH) on MRI. It is less clear if disruptions in cerebral blood flow caused by P.Hype can also contribute to a brain's small-vessel disease. For instance, microhemorrhages, especially if amyloid angiopathy co-occurs, may be precipitated by such sudden, overactive increases in orthostatic BP and, consequently, in the pressure of brain perfusion. Conversely, many neurodegenerative diseases may course with dysautonomia, including postural BP dysregulation. Lewy body disease (LBD) is the second most common neurodegenerative dementia (~ 20% of all dementia) and significant Lewy-body pathology co-occurs in approximately half of the cases diagnosed with Alzheimer's disease (AD) in post-mortem studies. Evidence is accumulating that AD, in its earliest stages, involves the brainstem. Since the neurovascular BP regulator control is located at the medulla oblongata, it is not surprising that many patients diagnosed with early-stage AD already have dysregulation in orthostatic BP control. Patients with Vascular Dementia (VD), which, together with LBD is the second most common dementing subtype, seem to have important impairment in the regulation of cerebral blood flow, especially if they also have unilateral or bilateral carotid stenosis greater than 50–70%. In patients with bilateral carotid stenosis greater than 70%, routine seated BP levels are inversely associated with ischemic strokes. Therefore, as exposed above, several lines of evidence point toward a vicious circle relationship between postural BP dysregulation and cognitive impairment/dementia. Since heart failure can contribute to P.Hypo, interventions that, in the long run, increase both the cardiac output and the neurocardiovascular tonus, such as aerobic exercise, may ameliorate P.Hypo. Moreover, dysregulation on the neurocardiovascular tonus, like that existent in overactive P.Hype, may also respond favorably to interventions that aim to improve both the cardiac function and the neurocardiovascular tonus, such as aerobic exercise.

1. Introduction

The cerebral autoregulation system allows maintenance of constant cerebral blood flow over a wide range of blood pressure. In old people, there is a progressive reshaping of cerebral autoregulation from a sigmoid curve to a straight line. This implies that any abrupt change in blood pressure will result in a rapid and significant change in cerebral blood flow [1].

Orthostatic hypotension (OH), however, is a common problem among older people, with a prevalence between 4% and 33%, depending on the methodology used and differences in population characteristics; this prevalence increases with age [2-4].

Although this variation may reflect true differences, discrepancies in prevalence may partly be due to methodological problems. Firstly, there are no uniform criteria in the medical literature as to the definition of OH, and a normal range of blood pressure change after standing in the elderly has not been established. Usually, OH is arbitrarily defined as a systolic blood pressure fall of more than 20 mmHg on standing, but when associated with relevant symptoms, indicating impaired cerebral perfusion, even a smaller drop in blood pressure may be of equal clinical importance [5].

Furthermore, the differences in prevalence may also be influenced by the selection of subjects, coexisting disorders, the use of medication associated with OH/hypotension and different methods for measuring OH. Many studies lack sufficient information about the basal supine-rest position which must precede the postural change [4].

It has been suggested that a resting period of at least 5±10 minutes is required to determine the stability or lack of stability of supine blood pressure. Moreover, in most reports, the blood pressure after standing has been measured for 1±3 minutes (or even just one measurement directly after standing). This might be a critical point in studies of OH, especially regarding prevalence, since this interval most certainly is not long enough [4].

Measurements of blood pressure in the standing position should be made preferably for a period of 10 min [5]. This suggestion is supported by our previous studies on dementia patients, where we found that 45% did not have their maximum systolic fall until 5 min or later [6]. Thus, the extent to which the prevalence of OH is reported in various study samples may, to a certain degree, be explained by methodological aspects [4].

Dementia is another common problem in elderly people. Worldwide, 25 million people suffer from dementia, the majority of whom have Alzheimer's disease (AD). It is a devastating illness, which results in a progressive decline in cognitive ability and functional capacity, causes immense distress to patients, their caregivers and families and has an enormous societal impact [7].

Despite the increasing prevalence of organic dementia with age, and the fact that OH is common among the elderly, very few studies have addressed the issue of whether OH may be a risk factor for developing dementia. In addition to the question of OH, few studies have investigated how hypotension as such might reflect cerebral circulation in patients with organic dementia [4].

Blood pressure (BP) abnormalities, both arterial hyper- and hypotension, as well as postural hypotension, have been reported in dementia both in clinical and neuropathological materials [4, 8-12]. Neuropathological studies have demonstrated that 50–60% of patients with AD also have selective incomplete white matter infarcts (SIWI) of a presumed ischemic etiology [13].

Hypotension and OH have previously also been recognized in about 40–50% of DLB cases and in a mixed DLB and AD population [13, 14]. Arterial hypotension may give rise to symptoms such as dizziness, loss of consciousness and syncope [15] as well as unsteady gait, falls and fractures [16, 17].

In addition, several commonly used drugs such as antihypertensives, diuretics, antidepressants, antianginal, neuroleptics and antiparkinson agents are known to yield hypotension and OH as a primary therapeutic effect or as an adverse effect [18-20].

Low BP and OH, which are common in organic dementia of all types (Passant et al., 1997) are suggested as an etiologic or as a complicating factor in dementia, particularly of the AD type [21, 22]. Previous hypertension that develops into hypotension, as well as other types of cardiac and vascular insufficiencies, have been suggested as contributing factors in dementia through the development of white matter infarcts [21, 23, 24]. It is suggested that episodes of hypoperfusion in a brain area due to BP falls, usually in combination with small vessel stenosis, results in complete and mainly incomplete white matter infarctions [9], particularly prevalent in the frontal lobes [21, 25].

Many recent studies observed among other data, that there was a correlation between systolic pressure reduction and cognitive decline, which was not accounted for by other factors. Some researchers speculate that blood pressure reduction might be an early change in the process of development of dementia. The most confounding factor is that low pressure by itself might be a predictor of death; nevertheless, the effect of low blood pressure on cognition is underestimated because of a survival bias [1].

Another explanation is that clinically unrecognized vascular lesions in the brain or atherosclerosis are responsible for both cognitive decline and blood pressure reduction. In particular, leuko-araiosis correlates with advancing age, cerebral atrophy, hypoperfusion of white matter, and cognitive impairments [26]. Leuko-araiosis is detectable in 9%–19% of older 'normal' subjects, but is virtually always present in vascular dementia (VaD). Leuko-araiosis, by itself, might be a risk factor for cognitive decline, as suggested in a recent study showing that normative subjects destined for later cognitive decline had excessive leuko-araiosis at study entry [26].

Thus, the researchers are trying to define the passage between normality, the so-called leuko-araiosis age-related and the excess of the response to the vascular damage, configuring the dementia, as a clinical syndrome. White matter injury may lead to brain atrophy or disrupted cholinergic fibers, but this relation has been incompletely studied [1].

Interestingly, the independent role of asymptomatic lacunar infarcts is less clear, with the possible exception of those involving the thalamus. Sensitive and specific definitions of cerebrovascular cognitive impairment are hampered by the fact that cerebrovascular disease is not easily linked to cognitive syndromes, either clinically or pathologically, and the presence of coincident Alzheimer disease (AD) is common [1].

Moreover, it is clear that some individuals may have a slowly progressive, dementing illness caused exclusively by cerebrovascular disease. Some individuals presenting cerebrovascular pathology probably have some component of AD pathology as part of their dementia; this relationship supports the possible interaction between cerebrovascular disease, aging, and the degenerative process [1].

Autonomic failure with orthostatic and postprandial hypotension, bowel and bladder disturbances, and sexual dysfunction are frequent, disabling features in patients with the three most prevalent neurodegenerative movement disorders: Parkinson's disease (PD), dementia with Lewy bodies and multiple system atrophy (MSA), and the related neurodegenerative Lewy-body disorder characterized by isolated severe autonomic failure (pure autonomic failure, PAF) [27].

All of these disorders have in common the presence of α-synuclein in the cytoplasmic precipitates found in neurons in Lewy body disorders or glia in MSA. Autonomic failure with disabling orthostatic hypotension is the clinical hallmark of PAF. It may also be the initial presentation of MSA, making diagnosis difficult. Within a few years, however, MSA patients develop movement disorders, which are differentiated from PD by the paucity of unilateral resting tremor, the lack of response to levodopa, and their rapidly progressive nature, resulting in disability and death in 7 to 8 years [27].

2. Age-Related Changes in Vascular Responses

The normal BP response that occurs when an individual moves from a supine to a standing position is a small reduction (<10 mm Hg) in SBP and a small increase in DBP (approximately 2.5 mm Hg). The hemodynamic response to an orthostatic reaction involves many organs. When a person stands up from a supine position, approximately 500 to 700 mL of blood is pooled in the lower extremities and in the splanchnic and pulmonary circulations. In response to the decrease in venous return to the heart, there is a transient reduction in cardiac output and stimulation of the baroreceptors, which reflexively increases sympathetic tone and vascular resistance and inhibits parasympathetic activity resulting in an increased heart rate [28].

Orthostatic hypotension is defined by the Consensus Committee of the American Autonomic Society and the American Academy of Neurology as a decline of >20 mm Hg in systolic blood pressure (SBP) or a decline of >10 mm Hg in diastolic blood pressure (DBP) that occurs when a person moves from a supine to a sitting or standing position. The decrease must be present within 3 minutes after the postural change [29].

Orthostatic hypotension can be asymptomatic, where BP changes occur without any symptoms or symptomatic, in which symptoms such as dizziness and faintness occur with BP changes. OH can also be classified into acute or reversible, typically caused by fluid volume loss or medication use and chronic or irreversible, caused by endocrine and neurogenic factors [28].

Normal aging is associated with an impaired ability for adaptation to environmental changes including impairment of the baroreflex. Thus, OH in older patients results from an excessive reduction in blood volume when patients are upright or from inadequate cardiovascular compensation. Changes in baroreceptor sensitivity, heart rate response, vascular compliance, vasopressin, renin, angiotensin, and renal concentrating abilities all contribute to increased risk for OH [28, 30].

Compliance and distensibility of the cardiovascular system diminish [31], as well as the cardiac output at supine rest [31, 32]. Blood volume and total red cell mass show a clear, although modest, reduction with age as does total volume of body fluids, which contributes to the relative deficiency of cardiovascular reflex regulation [33, 34].

Age is usually associated with changes in the cardiovascular system, especially in the structure and function of the arteries [35, 36]. Likewise, the risk of cardiovascular alterations is 2–5 times greater in elderly hypertensives than in normotensives of the same age [37], and two times more compared with younger patients with the same arterial pressure [38].

The cardiovascular alterations are responsible for 50% of morbidity and mortality in the elderly [39]. Both morbidity and mortality are dramatically increased when the aging process is associated with hypertension, which is a frequent pathology in this population [40]. In the elderly, cerebral perfusion is reduced, as a consequence of poor cerebral autoregulation associated with cerebral atherosclerosis, which alters both mental and physical functions; in addition, in patients with long-standing hypertension, the upper and lower limits of autoregulation tend to be shifted upwards [41], particularly in the elderly, so that even small decreases in blood pressure may induce significant reductions in cerebral blood flow [31].

Aging produces changes not only in vascular smooth muscle cells but also in endothelial cells[42]. The latter cells play a crucial role in vascular tone regulation [43; 44]. Different studies show that aging reduces the relaxations elicited by some vasodilators that release nitric oxide (NO) from endothelial cells [45-48].

Autonomic changes related to aging cause vasoconstriction, tachycardia and positive inotropy and lead to partial restoration of arterial pressure. A recent cross-sectional analysis of a population-based Cohort in the City of Kuopio, Finland investigated the postural changes in blood pressure and heart rate in elderly population. This study identified that OH-positive participants showed an increase of heart rate slightly more often than the OH-negative persons, whereas a minority of OH-negative persons maintained their BP by increasing the heart rate. This might indicate that reflex tachycardia is secondary in preventing an orthostatic reaction even in elderly persons. In addition, the heart rate changes in both the groups were minor, less than 10 beats per minute, which might suggest baroreflex impairment [49].

Pulse pressure in a supine position was higher in OH-positive than in OH-negative subjects. This can be explained by the fact that an increased resting pulse pressure indicates stiffness of the major arteries. Still, after rising to a standing position, the decrease of pulse pressure was also more pronounced in OH-positive than in OH-negative persons. The increased pulse pressure has been associated with a risk of major cardiovascular complications and mortality. However, the mean pressure is not the only factor resulting in a high cardiovascular risk in old patients [50].

Another important finding was that OH in elderly persons is independent of BP in sitting position and that diastolic OH after 1 min of standing was found to be more prevalent in the persons with low BP in a sitting position. This finding is notable because diastolic OH after 1 min predicted cardiovascular mortality in old persons.3 In addition, a diastolic BP drop, even when it is small enough not to fulfill the criteria of OH, after 1 min of standing up identifies the elderly persons at a high risk for myocardial infarction [51]. This might be due to the load the heart is exposed to upon rising up, and it may provoke coronary insufficiency and a decrease of stroke volume in frail elderly person [52].

3. Postural Blood Pressure Dysregulation in Age-Associated Neurological Disorders

3.1. Dementia and Blood Pressure Dysregulation

Regulation of the cerebrovascular system in dementia is a complex interplay between metabolic, chemical and neurogenic factors with the involvement of several neurotransmitters. The physiological basis of BP regulation involves both parasympathetic and sympathetic autonomic activity via the central cholinergic system [53]. Cerebral blood vessels are endowed with acetylcholinesterase positive fibers and It has been suggested that patients with impaired cholinergic function have a greater postural drop on standing and may also be the patients who will respond to cholinergic therapy [54].

An important study examined whether initially low blood pressure is related to the incidence of dementia in a sample of 304 persons, aged 75 to 96 years. The findings showed that compared with individuals with baseline systolic pressure of 140 to 179 mm Hg, those with systolic pressure of 140 mmHg or less had a significantly higher risk of dementia and AD. That was the first study to clearly report an association between relatively low systolic pressure and increased incidence of dementia [55].

Chronic low blood pressure has been positively associated with a number of clinical symptoms and psychosomatic distress – including unexplained fatigue, depression, and anxiety – and with minor psychiatric morbidity. A causal relationship between low blood pressure and low mood remains uncertain, but a vicious circle should not be excluded [56]. A correlation between systolic pressure reduction and cognitive decline in women, which was not accounted for by other factors, was observed in a community cohort of 924 elderly people with initially good cognition [57].

Blood pressure reduction might be an early change of the dementing process. An important study found that lower systolic and diastolic blood pressures at baseline were associated with a higher risk of dementia at follow-up. This association was observed across all age strata, in men as well in woman and both in AD and VaD. This may reflect that low blood pressure causes or contributes to dementia or that incipient dementia leads a drop in blood pressure [58].

In this study was observed an inverse association between blood pressure and dementia mainly in subjects, who used antihypertensive medication. This may indicate that their hypertension was longer lasting, and perhaps that these patients were more susceptible to pressure drops, causing inadequate cerebral blood flow. That would be particularly important in vulnerable areas, such as watershed zones and white matter [58].

On the other hand, low pressure might be a consequence of an incipient dementia. It was found that blood pressure was lower in subjects with manifest dementia, and those with dementia, who presented lower pressure, declined more rapidly. The possible explanation is that several areas are involved in pressure regulation [58].

Relatively low blood pressure seems to be correlated with dementia even in a preclinical stage. Guo and colleagues (1999) started from the speculation that cerebral blood flow is reduced in dementia patients [55, 59]. That was generally thought to be related with reduced metabolic activity of the brain or with a major vascular lesion. The authors hypothesized that the reduction of cerebral blood flow might be related to the impairment of the cerebral autoregulation, secondary to the degenerative disorder. The direct consequence would be a sequential ulterior reduction of blood pressure, due to dysregulation, which might accelerate the lowering of blood perfusion and therefore the underlying degenerative process [22, 60-63]. Lower systolic blood pressure was associated with cognitive decline and dementia. Earlier history of arterial hypertension was related to an increased risk of impaired cognition and dementia. Nilsson and colleagues (2007) [63] interpreted these results as a potential expression of the frailty and deteriorated vitality of the oldest elderly, in keeping constantly the autoregulation capabilities of the normal brain, and expressed their concern, due to this frailty, on the real impact of lowering pressure in oldest age [1].

There is strong evidence of a cerebral cholinergic defect in patients with dementia including the most common causes of dementia like AD, LBD and VaD [25]. The importance of the dopaminergic system has been more emphasised in relation to neuropharmacological issues than to cerebrovascular physiology. However, a recent study [64] found that blood vessels in the mesencephalon change in patients with Parkinson's disease and the authors suggested that modifications in the microenvironment of dopaminergic neurones may be important in the pathogenesis of brain diseases. The larger number of neuroleptics prescribed for patients with dementia is probably other important factor for the high prevalence of OH in this group [25].

The effect of standing up on blood pressure and pulse reaction is important to clarify for several reasons. First, it might be used as an instrument to differentiate different types of dementia from each other. This will have clinical implications as DLB patients show good responsiveness to cholinesterase inhibitors but extreme sensitivity to the side effects of neuroleptic drugs. It is also important since the course and prognosis may differ from other dementias [65]. Second, it is important to recognise a low blood pressure in patients with dementia as many of the drugs used to treat dementia have blood pressure lowering properties and specific interventions may be necessary to improve related symptoms and reduce the risk of falls [7].

It is important to test for OH during 10 min of standing since patients, and dementia patients in particular, may not manifest significant falls in blood pressure until after five minutes of standing or more [6].

3.2. Alzheimer's Disease

Alzheimer's disease (AD) is a complex neurodegenerative disease characterized by impairment in cognitive function, behavior and ability to perform activities of daily living. Both neurochemical and neurohistological alterations contribute to the clinical manifestations in patients with AD. The disease is associated with progressive neuronal loss in the association and limbic areas of the cerebral cortex, and in the basal forebrain cholinergic system [66]. Areas of the prefrontal and anterior cingulated cortex, medial temporal and the basal forebrain, have intimate connections with the nuclei controlling autonomic function [67].

The cholinergic system originates in the forebrain and projects diffusely to the cerebral cortex. In AD, there is a marked loss of neurons in the basal forebrain nuclei, which usually exceeds 75% of the total neuronal population at the time of an autopsy [68; 69]. The death of cholinergic neurons leads to reductions in choline acetyltransferase in the hippocampus and temporal cortex [68, 70]. There is also an overall loss in acetylcholinesterase (AChE) in the brains of patients with AD [70, 71].

The loss of central cholinergic activity has been correlated with severity of dementia on dementia rating scales [72]. On the basis of these findings, it has been hypothesized that the deficit in cholinergic transmission plays a primary role in the pathogenesis of AD [73]. Currently available AD-specific therapies include a symptomatic approach based on enhancement of cholinergic function [74].

In addition, hypotension after a meal is greater in AD patients than in healthy elderly subjects. Postprandial BP in the elderly depends on hemodynamics, autonomic and hormonal changes related to meal-induced splanchnic blood pooling [75]. Sympathetic vasomotor dysfunction [76] and BP instability of central origin [77] have been reported in AD. It is impossible to exclude an abnormal cardiac vasomotor response that is unmasked by food ingestion [78].

There is some evidence that factors independent of autonomic regulation are involved in heart rate changes after food [75]. The heart rate increases in the AD patients and in the elderly control subjects were not related to the degree of postprandial hypotension. The maximum BP fall in AD occurred after the first hour after food ingestion, in contrast to chronic autonomic failure, where it occurs soon after meals [79]. Different postprandial hypotension mechanisms could be involved in AD. It is important to consider the potential clinical implications of postprandial hypotension in AD patients; these include falls, confusion and temporary worsening of cognitive deficits [78].

The possible association of vascular mechanisms and the development of AD have been a recent topic of discussion. It has been suggested that vascular factors are important contributory factors in AD [80]. White matter disease is frequently found in the brains of AD [9]. The most marked white matter changes typical of AD, constitute a combination of axonal and myelin reduction, a mild reactive gliosis and a small vessel arteriosclerosis. Described as selective incomplete white matter infarction [81] these changes are considered to be ischemic/vascular in type, albeit generally associated with the primary neurodegenerative disease of AD [82].

Cerebral amyloid angiopathy, however, in itself a vascular disorder directly associated with AD, has no immediate association with traditional cerebrovascular disease factors, such as atherosclerosis, hypertension and hyperlipidemia [83], but has been shown to correlate with severity of white matter disease [84]. This type of disease, judged to be a form of vascular ischemic complication in many AD patients, occurs and progresses along the course of dementia [85, 86]. Although cerebral amyloid angiopathy in AD correlates positively with white matter disease severity, the former is also more prevalent in higher ages. These correlations indicate a multifatorial pathogenesis of white matter disease in AD, in which other vascular and/or cardiac features may possibly play a role [82].

In clinical dementia research hypertension and orthostatic hypotension are frequently investigated features [4, 87-89], and an association between elevated blood pressure and white matter lesions is recognized [90-94]. Recently, a study had found that hypertension as well as orthostatic hypotension were more frequent in AD with white matter disease than in AD without white matter disease. Earlier studies have shown that midlife hypertension increases the risk of AD in later life [95; 96]. These latter studies, however, had no neuropathological confirmation of the clinical diagnoses, or reference to any coexisting white matter disease [82].

Previous studies, however, have shown that variability in blood pressure has a stronger correlation to white matter disease than hypertension per se [89; 97]. One may speculate that a lack of capacity to regulate abnormal blood pressure, well recognized in AD [98], leads to recurrent dysfunction of cerebral perfusion and leaves room for the development of white matter disease [99].

3.3. Vascular Dementia

Vascular Dementia (VaD) refers to a broad category of patients, where a multi-faceted cognitive decline is attributed to cerebrovascular disease. It lists different pathologies, in order to identify patients with different subtypes of VaD: multi-infarct dementia (multiple large and complete infarcts), post-hemorrhage dementia, and subcortical VaD, a small vessel disease [1].

Subcortical VaD (sVaD) is mainly due to lacunar infarct, occurring in distribution of small arterioles, usually in the white matter, basal ganglia, thalamus and pons, or to microinfarct – not seen on macroscopic examination – a small area of cystic or noncystic necrosis surrounded by astrocytes. Incomplete infarct may also be present, due to a selective loss of neurons, myelin, and oligodendrocytes, without cystic necrosis, occurring in the periphery of major artery distribution infarcts (eg, penumbra) or in deep white matter. Incomplete White matter infarcts are associated with myelin pallor, astrocytosis, and a variable degree of axonal loss [1].

Subcortical VaD now incorporates the old entities of 'lacunar state' and 'Binswanger's disease', and it relates to small vessel disease and hypoperfusion, resulting in focal and diffuse ischaemic white matter lesions and incomplete ischaemic injury [100, 101]. Small vessel dementia is presumably the most frequently pathological condition observed in elderly patients [102]. It is due to infarcts caused by obstruction of intracerebral vessels of arteriolar size, subcortically represented by the long penetrant arteries. The cause may be micro-emboli from heart valves or atheromatous large vessel lesions, particularly carotid stenosis or special vessel diseases such as collagen or inflammatory diseases [103], amyloid angiopathy, and other hereditary angiopathies [1].

The major known causative factor of VaD is hypertensive angiopathy. It may assume two forms: cortical plus subcortical, and purely subcortical, referred to as Binswanger's disease or progressive subcortical vascular encephalopathy. The lacunar state may be regarded as a milder form of the latter. The two varieties are basically similar, showing mostly small infarcts of lacunar size up to 10 to 15 mm in diameter [104]. Binswanger's disease is marked by lacunar infarcts usually measuring 5–10 mm in diameter and situated in the brain stem and central gray nuclei but above all in the frontal white matter, sparing the cortex and u-fibers. In the white matter the lacunes are surrounded by wide areas of incomplete infarcts with partial loss of axons, myelin and oligodendroglial cells accompanied by a mild astrocytic gliosis causing an extensive cortical undermining and disconnection [1].

This change impresses as the main structural substrate for the functional deficit in Binswanger's disease, explaining, for example, frontal symptoms, gait, and incontinence problems. The small lacunes are probably of lesser importance. The loss of white matter is reflected in a widening of especially the frontal ventricular horns. Portions of less severe incomplete white matter infarcts may not be demonstrable on brain imaging, causing clinical-pathological correlation difficulties [104, 105].

Hypertension has often been observed to be a risk factor for VaD [106-108] and sometimes for AD [109-11]. Hypertension leads to changes in arterioles and eventually to arteriolar occlusive disease and then on to infarction. Hypertension's effects on the brain in VaD or AD could also be related to changes in blood flow or blood-brain-barrier integrity. A large number of epidemiological studies show strong associations between elevations in middle-life blood pressure and the prevalence of later life cognitive impairment and dementia. Early evidence suggest that treatment hypertension in the elderly may be quite successful in reducing incident dementia [1].

In the Syst-Eur trial [112], cognition was primarily assessed by the Mini-Mental State Examination. Treatment with a calcium channel blocking antihypertensive was associated with a nearly 50% reduction in incident dementia amongst approximately 2000 elderly with isolated systolic hypertension. The conclusions of this study, given the high percentage of elderly suffering with untreated hypertension, are that secondary prevention treatment trials such as Syst-Eur might have a substantial impact on cognitive impairment [1].

The relation between hypertension, its treatment, and severe white matter lesions has been assessed in 10 European cohorts [89]. White matter lesions in the periventricular and subcortical regions were rated separately using semiquantitative measures. Increase in systolic blood pressure levels were associated with more severe periventricular and subcortical white matter lesions. People with poorly controlled hypertension had a higher risk of severe white matter lesions than those without hypertension [89].

Recent works, however, underline a potential negative effect by decreasing diastolic blood pressure level on the occurrence of severe periventricular white matter lesions. A high pulse pressure is related to arterial stiffness, which might be considered one of its clinical indicator, and it is associated with an increased risk of dementia [113]. Therefore, it could be postulated that functional changes of the arterial system are involved in the pathogenesis of dementia [1].

The traditional general practice teaches that "the lower the blood pressure is, the better the prognosis". Albeit this, low blood pressure as a predictor of increased mortality has been described in a 5-year prospective study in Finland [114] as well as paradoxical survival of elderly men with high blood pressure [115]. Interpretations of these so-called J-shaped curves between blood pressure, and mortality have always been viewed with caution and skepticism by epidemiologists and statisticians [116, 117].

Anatomically, the smaller resistance blood vessels undergo degenerative changes consisting of thickening and fibrosis of the media and intima, and patchy degeneration of smooth muscle cells producing luminal narrowing and increased vascular resistance. Although the resting cerebral blood flow is the same in normotensive and hypertensive individuals, these structural changes limit the capacity of the resistance vessels for maximal vasodilatation. These changes also impair tolerance of lower blood pressures, while improving tolerance to hypertension through vasoconstriction of these same vessels [1].

The prevalence of orthostatic and nonorthostatic hypotension reached 50% in clinically evaluated VaD cases [118; 119]. The possible reason that relates lower blood pressure, dysregulation of cerebral blood flow and vascular dementia, is the pivotal role of acetylcholine (ACh). ACh regulates the cerebral blood flow through the parasympathetic innervations of the circle of Willis and of the pial vessels [120], and it causes significant arterial relaxation by promoting the synthesis of vasodilator agents [121]. In humans, post-mortem studies have shown that choline acetyltransferase (ChAT) activity is reduced in VaD patients, compared with controls [122].

Furthermore, clinical studies have indicated that patients with subcortical VaD have significantly lower concentrations of ACh in the cerebrospinal fluid, and that these decreases are strongly correlated with cognitive deficits [122]. The number of muscarinic cholinergic receptors is also markedly reduced in VaD and mixed dementia patients [123]. In addition, the level of ACh in the cerebral fluid of VaD patients is significantly lower than in controls, but is similar to the level observed in AD patients [124].

Therefore, it might be hypothesized that the damage of arteriole causes a reduction of cerebral blood flow. The other macroscopic consequence is the disruption of the cerebral autoregulation. The dysregulation is augmented by the reduction of ACh. These aspects might determine the sensitiveness of old patients, and especially demented patients, to hypotension. Each clinical condition that may lead to hypotension might accelerate the underlying degenerative process [1].

3.4. Dementia of Lewy Bodies

The Lewy body syndromes may affect peripheral autonomic, brain-stem, basal ganglia, and cortical neurons. Lewy bodies are intracytoplasmic neuronal inclusions that contain abnormally phosphorylated intermediate neurofilament proteins, α-synuclein, ubiquitin, and associated enzymes [27].

It is likely that the clinical phenotype of Lewy body syndromes depends on the temporal formation and distribution of Lewy bodies and associated neurodegeneration. In Pure Autonomic Failure (PAF), there is early and widespread involvement of peripheral autonomic neurons. In Parkinson's Disease (PD) there is neuronal loss in the substantia nigra and other brain-stem nuclei, and in DLB there is cortical involvement. Individual differences in neuronal susceptibility may determine the presenting phenotype. Patients with PAF, however, can progress to PD or Dementia with Lewy bodies (DLB) [27], suggesting that phenotypes overlap and that neurodegeneration in the Lewy body syndromes may start in postganglionic autonomic neurons and later affect neurons in the central nervous system (CNS) [27].

DLB is often claimed to be the second most common cause of neurodegenerative dementia in older people after AD. A systematic review of six studies has found prevalence estimates for clinical DLB of up to 30.5% of all dementia cases [125].

The central feature of DLB is progressive cognitive decline accompanied by fluctuating cognition, visual hallucinations and parkinsonism. Suggestive features are REM sleep behaviour disorder, severe neuroleptic sensitivity and low dopamine transporter uptake in basal ganglia. Some of the supportive features are falls, syncope, loss of consciousness, systematized delusions, hallucinations of other modalities, depression, autonomic failure and abnormal metaiodobenzyl guanidine (MIBG) myocardial scintigraphy [126-128].

The most common autonomic symptom in DLB is orthostatic intolerance. Compared to PD, the frequency of orthostatic intolerance was greater in DLB but was comparable to Multiple System Atrophy (MSA). The severity of this set of symptoms varied widely in DLB, again positioning this group in between the more severe symptoms of MSA and the milder ones in PD. Most

MSA patients with orthostatic symptoms needed medications while most DLB patients responded to volume expansion alone. When the DLB patients were treated, they responded better to medications than MSA patients, providing support that the autonomic deficits were less severe overall [27].

Autonomic function, however, such as OH has not been adequately studied in DLB, although preliminary reports indicate that it is a major problem in these patients [65]. DLB patients had a greater drop in blood pressure during orthostatic challenge over 10 min, than patients with AD or elderly controls. Furthermore was reported an important finding, demonstrating that DLB patients had a significantly more protracted period of orthostasis than AD patients. The pulse drive was similar in DLB and AD, but the rise in pulse rate was not adequate to restore the blood pressure to supine values in DLB patients. There is also a significantly higher prevalence of OH in patients suffering from dementia compared to older people without dementia [7].

The profile of the orthostatic reaction is different between dementia groups. DLB has the greatest drop in blood pressure and most longstanding reaction to orthostatic challenge. This may have clinical implications for treatment as well as for understanding the neurophysiological properties of the disease. Further studies are needed to determine if OH can play a more important role in the diagnosis of DLB [7].

3.5. Parkinson's Disease

Orthostatic hypotension (OH) occurs commonly in Parkinson's disease (PD) [129, 130], often exacerbated by the hypotensive effect of dopaminergic drugs [131]. Neuropathological correlates of OH in PD include Lewy Body (LB) degeneration in sympathetic ganglia [132]. The Braak staging of Parkinson's disease emphasizes early involvement of the brainstem, including the dorsal vagal nucleus, and autonomic failure is a feature of Parkinson's disease [133].

In a study of 116 patients with typical PD by clinical criteria, almost two thirds had orthostatic hypotension with symptoms of cerebral hypoperfusion, including syncope, when tested in a tilt table for 40 minutes or until symptoms developed [134].

Other study found a fall of at least 20 mm Hg of systolic blood pressure was found in almost 60% of patients with PD with OH symptomatic in 20% of the patients [129]. It was related to duration and severity of the disease and with the use of higher daily levodopa and bromocriptine doses [129]. Vagal control of the heart and hemodynamic response to standing were impaired and related to duration of symptoms of PD [135].

Dysautonomia in PD, however, appears to be less common and mild than in dementia with Lewy Bodies (DLB) reflecting more extensive LB pathology in DLB [130, 136]. Whether OH is also common in PD with delayed dementia (PDD) has not been investigated systematically, however, the widespread DLB-like neuropathology of PDD suggests that dysautonomia may be more common in this disorder compared to PD [137].

Similarly, autonomic dysfunction in PD is rarely as severe as in patients with MSA. In most cases, autonomic failure occurs late, but there is a subgroup of PD patients with clinically significant autonomic failure early in the course of the disease. The confounding effect of antiparkinsonian medication, which frequently worsens orthostatic hypotension, and difficulties in the differential diagnosis, particularly between PD and MSA, make it difficult to estimate accurately the prevalence of autonomic dysfunction in patients with PD. Studies may overestimate the frequency of autonomic dysfunction in PD if they mistakenly include patients with MSA or underestimate it if PD patients with autonomic dysfunction are diagnosed as MSA [137].

Fluctuating attention is also frequently present in PDD patients [126]. Its underlying substrate is unclear, however, disturbances of cholinergic transmission are likely to contribute [138]. Whether impaired regulation of orthostatic blood pressure exacerbates attentional deficits in PDD has not been addressed, although several studies suggest a correlation between impaired cognitive performance and OH [3, 139].

Recently was demonstrated that OH occurs more frequently and more severely in PDD than in PD patients and exacerbates attentional deficits. OH may also be related to the occurrence of transient fluctuations in attention observed in PDD patients [140], consistent with the general notion of cognitive failure resulting from chronic arterial hypotension [131, 141].

Considering that OH was associated with cerebral hypoperfusion and accumulation of amyloid beta protein in cortical arterial boundary zones and other areas susceptible to ischemia in postmortem study with PDD patients [142], these patients may be at higher risk of entering a vicious circle where the autonomic failure produces OH which favors the occurrence of degenerative lesions, aggravating the autonomic dysfunction and worsening the course of the disease [137].

3.6. Multiple System Atrophy

MSA is a rare and progressive neurodegenerative disorder of unknown cause affecting extrapyramidal, pyramidal, cerebellar, and autonomic pathways. This disease included the disorders previously called striatonigral degeneration (SND, with predominant movement disorders), sporadic olivopontocerebellar atrophy (OPCA, with predominant cerebellar symptoms), and the Shy-Drager syndrome (SDS, with predominant autonomic symptoms) [143]. Data shows a prevalence of 4.4/ 100,000 and an incidence of 3/100,000 per year [144; 145].

The discovery of glial cytoplasmic inclusions (GCIs) in the brains of patients with MSA provided a pathological marker for the disorder and confirmed that SND, OPCA, and SDS are one disease with different clinical expressions [146]. The lesion resides within the CNS and impairs the neural connections responsible for baroreflex modulation of sympathetic tone. On the other hand, the neurons that tonically discharge sympathetic activity (e.g., those residing in the rostral ventrolateral medulla or in the spinal cord) and distal pathways (e.g., spinal tracts and postganglionic noradrenergic fibers) appear to be intact in MSA [27].

The disease can cause Parkinsonism, cerebellar, pyramidal, autonomic, and urological dysfunction in any combination [147]. Most patients are in their early 50s, with men more commonly affected than women (ratio of 1.3:1). The initial clinical presentation can be either autonomic or motor deficits. When the initial deficit is autonomic, it is usually the symptoms of orthostatic hypotension, either lightheadedness or syncope, that send the afflicted patient to the physician. Postprandial hypotension, bowel and bladder motility disturbances, and sexual and thermoregulatory dysfunctions quickly become apparent. The initial clinical presentation of these patients may resemble PAF, making a definite diagnosis difficult early in the disease process [27].

Within 5 years, but usually less, most patients with MSA who had autonomic deficits at the onset of their illness show motor symptoms. In some patients, their illness appears to begin with motor rather than autonomic deficits. In 80% of patients with MSA, the predominant motor deficit is

Parkinsonism with progressive akinesia and rigidity, postural tremor, and less frequently resting tremor. Because Parkinsonism is the most frequent motor deficit in MSA patients, these patients are often misdiagnosed as suffering PD [148].

Asymmetrical symptoms are not infrequent. In 20% of patients, cerebellar deficits predominate with gait and limb ataxia, pronounced scanning dysarthria, and oculomotor abnormalities [148]. Late in the disease, cerebellar and Parkinsonian deficits can be combined, but clinical recognition of cerebellar deficits may be difficult when pronounced parkinsonism is present. Half of the patients have pyramidal signs and severe dementia is most unusual [148, 149].

3.7. Huntington's Disease

Huntington's disease (HD) is an autosomal dominant degenerative neurologic disorder of the central nervous system (CNS) characterized by a classical triad of symptoms, including involuntary movements, behavioral abnormalities, personality changes, and cognitive impairment. Previous studies have shown Autonomic Nervous System (ANS) hypofunction in HD patients, and attributed it to a diminished input from higher centers to the intact brainstem sympathetic system [150; 151]. It has also been suggested that the central autonomic network function declines as the disease progresses [151].

In addition, a recent study confirmed that heart rate variability (HRV) indices decline in HD patients overall [152]. However, reduced vagal modulation of HRV and relative sympathetic predominance was found in mid-stage HD patients according to the motor function subscale of the United Huntington disease rating scale (UHDRS) [152]. Nevertheless, cardiovascular ANS function in asymptomatic gene carriers as a separate group has not been evaluated yet [153].

A recent study have shown that mild sympathetic hyperactivity is present already in asymptomatic gene carriers and is even more pronounced in mildly disabled HD patients. Advanced HD is associated with predominantly parasympathetic dysfunction. Deficient parasympathetic activity in HD patients is indicated by a drop in HRV during forced ventilation, and by a lesser increase in heart rate on standing up. This is in accordance with findings in a previous study [151]. These findings suggest that ANS is one of the early affected neuronal systems not only in HD patients but also in asymptomatic HD gene carriers [153].

4. Management

Treatment of OH should be individualized. Often, treatment is implemented in order to improve functional capacity and sense of well-being rather than to reach a fixed value of arterial pressure. The goal of treatment is to make the patient symptom-free and able to walk without dizziness or lightheadedness.

Patients need to maintain adequate fluid intake, limit or avoid alcohol, and exercise regularly in the horizontal position (e.g., swimming and bed exercises such as moving feet up and down to activate calf muscle pump). It is recommendable to change posture slowly and avoid standing still. When standing for a prolonged time, they should cross and uncross the legs a few times in order to increase venous return [28].

Patients on prolonged bed rest need to slowly increase the amount of time they spend seated each day. Fitted elastic hose or compression stockings may enhance cardiac output and standing BP, thereby reducing venous pooling in the legs. Hose or stockings must be worn all day in order to be useful [28].

They need to eat small meals frequently and avoid standing up suddenly after eating. It is also important to avoid hot showers or excessive heat and also to avoid straining during micturition and defecation. Patients without hypertension need to increase salt intake [28].

Low levels of exercise may be helpful but this needs careful consideration, since activities which involve straining may also increase the orthostatic reactions, particularly in patients with autonomic dysfunction [154]. Oral caffeine, preferably given before breakfast, may be effective and particularly prevent postprandial hypotension [155]. The ideal agent or agents to control unwanted hypotension has not yet been identified. This is complicated by the fact that many drugs may produce different hemodynamic responses in different patients [4].

Patients should exercise the calf muscles before sitting up, and sit on the edge of the bed for a few minutes before standing to give the body time to adjust to the postural change and help the blood flow back to the heart [28].

Patients should avoid bending at the waist to pick up items from the floor or to reach for something on a lower shelf. If possible, squat at the knees and keep the head above the level of the heart. Consider wearing waist-length elastic stockings to prevent venous pooling in the legs. Use a urinal or bedside commode to reduce the need to get up quickly or rely on assistance in order to use the bathroom [156].

Orthostatic hypotension is often successfully treated with fludrocortisone and oral adrenergic vasoconstrictors like midodrine [157, 158]. Reversing the anemia common in patients with MSA using recombinant erythropoietin increases upright blood pressure and ameliorates symptoms of orthostatic hypotension [159, 160].

The elderly may be especially vulnerable to side-effects, because of complicating disorders and age-related physiological changes, which increase their sensitivity to medication. Drug therapy (i.e., fluorocortisone and sympatho-mimetic amines) may be effective [161, 162]. Unfortunately, side-effects often limit use, and all pharmacological treatment has to be used with great caution in the elderly, especially in demented patients, who might not be able to communicate and report such side-effects [4].

Recent evidence suggests that ventricular hypertrophy develops in hypertensive patients with autonomic failure [163], and that there are many cases of fatal strokes in these patients. During the daytime, effective treatment of supine hypertension can be easily accomplished simply by avoiding the supine position. Sleeping in the head-up tilt position reduces nocturnal sodium loss, which will improve orthostatic hypotension in the morning [164, 165]. This approach, however, is often insufficient to treat supine hypertension [27].

The Epicardian Study (an examination of 2,700 patients age >65) found that adequate control of blood pressure itself reduces the incidence of OH associated with hypertension [166]. Changes in frequency of OH before and after treatment of hypertension suggest that lowering blood pressure adequately with treatment decreases the prevalence of OH [167].

Antihypertensives that can cause OH, such as diuretics, alpha blockers and central alpha agonists, may be replaced by agents that are associated with a lower frequency of OH. These include beta-adrenergic agonists, angiotensin converting enzyme (ACE) inhibitors, and selected calcium channel blockers. OH may be seen with beta blockers that have some alpha–blocking properties, such as labetalol. The reported prevalence of OH with labetalol is 1.4%.12 A comparison of enalapril (5 to 20 mg/d) with long-acting nifedipine (30 to 90 mg/d) found enalapril reduces the number of OH episodes, whereas long-acting nifedipine increases the phenomenon [168].

In movement disorders, moderately effective treatment is available for autonomic symptoms, but management of movement disorders by itself remains unsuccessful [27]. Discoveries relevant to physiology and common pathological conditions were initially made in patients with autonomic failure. Meals induce profound hypotension in these patients. Conversely, commonly used nasal decongestants can produce substantial pressor effects. Even 500 mL of water can increase blood pressure by a previously unrecognized sympathetic reflex. Residual sympathetic tone is able to induce sustained supine hypertension in MSA, because it is resolved after ganglionic blockade. These phenomena were not previously recognized because of the buffering capacity of the baroreflex, but were unmasked in autonomic failure patients [27].

5. Conclusions

The increased frequency of autonomic neuropathy, especially the high prevalence of orthostatic hypotension emphasizes the importance of these conditions in all people with dementia. Their impact on key symptoms such as dizziness, syncope, falls, constipation and incontinence needs to be investigated—although orthostatic blood pressure responses can be impaired for a number of other reasons, including medications, endothelial dysfunction and age-related orthostatic hypotension.

It is important to highlight the role of orthostatic hypotension in all patients with dementia and the need for further research into sustained orthostatic hypotension as a modifiable risk factor for falls. In elderly people, simple measures such as adequate hydration, support hosiery and pharmacological treatments such as fludrocortisone and midodrine can be used to manage orthostatic hypotension, as part of a multifactorial intervention to reduce the risk of falls [169].

Cholinergic dysfunction has been discussed as a potential cause of autonomic failure in patients with dementia, and may be particularly important in PDD and DLB, where cholinergic deficits are especially pronounced, and where the disease pathology involves the dorsal vagal nucleus [133].

Aging also affects the cardiovascular responses to changes in posture. Older subjects have been found to have lower heart rate responses to orthostatic stress than the young [170, 171]. Chronic exercise training can affect these cardiovascular responses to submaximal orthostatic stress in older adults [171, 172]. Physical activity has been associated with an attenuation in the reduction in resting cerebral blood flow [173], suggesting that exercise may have a beneficial effect in the elderly [174].

References

[1] Moretti, R; Torre, P; Antonello, RM; Manganaro, D; Vilotti, C; Pizzolato, G. Risk factors for vascular dementia: hypotension as a key point. *Vasc Health Risk Manag*. 2008; 4 (2):395-402.

[2] Mathias, CJ; Kimber JR. Postural hypotension: causes, clinical features, investigation, and management. *Annu Rev Med*. 1999b; 50: 317–336.

[3] Kenny, RA; Kalaria, R; Ballard, C. Neurocardiovascular instability in cognitive impairment and dementia. *Ann N Y Acad Sci*. 2002; 977: 183–195.

[4] Passant, U; Warkentin S; Gustafson l. Orthostatic hypotension and low blood pressure in organic dementia: a study of prevalence and related clinical characteristics. *Int J Geriatr Psychiatry,* 1997; 12: 395-403.

[5] Mathias, CJ; Bannister, R. Investigation of autonomic disorders. In: *Autonomic Failure. A Text-book of Clinical Disorders of the Autonomic Nervous System*, 3rd ed. (R. Bannister and C. J. Mathias, Eds). Oxford University Press, Oxford, 1992a. pp. 255-290.

[6] Passant, U; Warkentin, S; Karlson, S; Nilsson, K; Edvinsson, L; Gustafson, L. Orthostatic hypotension in organic dementia: Relationship between blood pressure, cortical blood flow and symptoms. *Clin. Auton. Res*. 1996; 6: 29-36.

[7] Andersson, M; Hansson, O; Minthon, L; Ballard, CG; Londos, E. The period of hypotension following orthostatic challenge is prolonged in dementia with Lewy bodies. *Int J Geriatr Psychiatry*, 2008; 23: 192–198.

[8] Brun, A; Englund, E. White matter changes in Alzheimer's presenile and senile dementia. In: Gottfries, C.G. (Ed.), *Normal Aging,*

Alzheimer's disease and Senile Dementia. Editions de l'Universite´ de Bruxelles, Bruxelles, 1985. pp. 47–50.

[9] Brun, A; Englund, E. A white matter disorder in dementia of the Alzheimer type: a pathoanatomical study. *Ann. Neurol*. 1986; 19: 253–262.

[10] Sulkava, R; Erkinjuntti, T. Vascular dementia due to cardiac arrytmias and systemic hypotension. *Acta Neurol. Scand*. 1987; 76: 123–128.

[11] Erkinjuntti, T; Hachinski, VC. Rethinking vascular dementia. *Cerebrovasc. Disord*. 1993; 3: 3–23.

[12] Wallin, A; Blennow, K. Heterogeneity of vascular dementia. Mechanisms and subgroups. *J.Geriatr. Psychiatry*. 1993; 6: 137–145.

[13] Kuzuhara, S; Yoshimura, M; Mizutani, T; Yamanouchi, H. Clinical features of diffuse Lewy body disease in the elderly: analysis of 12 cases. In: Perry, R., McKeith, I., Perry, E. (Eds.), *Dementia with Lewy Bodies — Clinical, Pathological and Treatment Issues*. Cambridge University Press, UK, 1996. pp. 153–160.

[14] Ballard, CG; Shaw, F; Lowery, K; McKeith, I; Kenny, R. The prevalence, assessment and associations of falls in dementia with Lewy bodies and Alzheimer's disease. *Dement. Geriatr. Cogn. Disord*. 1999; 10: 97–103.

[15] Bradshaw, MJ; Edwards, RTM. Postural hypotension—pathophysiology and management. *Q.J. Med*. 1986; 231: 643–657.

[16] Rubenstein, LZ; Robbins, AS. Falls in the elderly a clinical approach. *Geriatria* 1984; 39: 67–78.

[17] Tinetti, ME; Williams, TF; Mayewski, R. Fallrisk index for elderly patients based on the number of chronic disabilities. *Am. J. Med*. 1986; 80: 429–434.

[18] Schoenberger, JA. Drug-induced orthostatic hypotension. *Drug Saf*. 1991; 6: 402–407.

[19] McCarthy, P; Cameron, S. Orthostatic hypotension: a potential side effects of psychiatric medicaitons. *J. Psychosoc. Nurs*. 1992; 30: 3–5.

[20] Mets, TF. Drug-induced orthostatic hypotension in older patients. *Drugs Aging*. 1995; 6: 219–228.

[21] Englund, E; Brun, A; Gustafson, L. A white matter disease in dementia of Alzheimer's type—clinical and neuropathological correlates. *Int. J. Geriatr. Psychiatry* 1989; 4: 87–102.

[22] Guo, Z; Viitanen, M; Fratiglioni, L; Winblad, B. Low blood pressure and dementia in elderly people: the Kungsholmen project. *Br. Med. J.* 1996; 312: 805–808.

[23] Skoog, I; Lernfeldt, B; Landahl, S; Palmertz, B; Andreasson, LA; Nilsson, L; Persson, G; Ode′n, A; Svanborg, A. 15-Year longitudinal study of blood pressure and dementia. *Lancet* 1996; 347: 1141–1145.

[24] Englund, E. 1999. Neuropathology of white matter disease: parenchymal changes. In: Pantoni, L., Inzitari, D., Wallin A. (Eds.), *Clinical and Patholphysiological Aspects of White Matter Disease Related to Cognitive Decline and Vascular Dementia,* ICG Publications, Dordrecht, The Netherlands, in press.

[25] Londos, E; Passant, U; Gustafson, L. Blood pressure and drug treatment in clinically diagnosed Lewy body dementia and Alzheimer's disease. *Archives of Gerontology and Geriatrics.* 2000; 30: 35–46.

[26] Meyer, JS; Rauch, G; Rauch, RA; et al. Risk factors for cerebral hypoperfusion, mild cognitive impairment, and dementia. *Neurobiol Aging*, 2000; 21:161–169.

[27] Kaufmann, H; Biaggioni, I. Autonomic Failure in Neurodegenerative Disorders. *Seminars in Neurology*. 2003; 23 (4): 351-363.

[28] Sclater, A; Alagiakrishnan, K. Orthostatic hypotension A primary care primer for assessment and treatment. *Geriatrics August*. 2004 (8): 22-27.

[29] Consensus statement on the definition of orthostatic hypotension, pure autonomic failure, and multiple system atrophy. The Consensus Committee of the American Autonomic Society and the American Academy of Neurology. *Neurology* 1996; 46(5):1470.

[30] Roth, GS. Hormone/neurotransmitter action during aging: the calcium hypothesis of impaired signal transduction. *Rev. Biol. Res. Aging*. 1990; 4: 243-252.

[31] Folkow, B; Svanborg, A. Physiology of vascular aging. *Physiol. Rev.* 1993; 73: 725-764.

[32] Brandfonbrener, M; Landowne, M; Shock, NW. Changes in cardiac output with age. *Circulation*, 1955; 12: 557-565.

[33] Messerli, FH; Sungaard-Riise, K; Ventura, HO; Dunn, FG; Glade, LB; Frohlich, ED. Essential hypertension in the elderly: haemodynamics. intravascular volume, plasma renin activity, and circulating catecholamine levels. *Lancet*, 1983; 2: 983-986.

[34] Messerli, FH. Essential hypertension in the elderly. Triangle. 1985; 24: 35-47.

[35] Wei, JY. Use of calcium entry blockers in elderly patients, *Circulation*. 1989; 80: IV-171-IV-177.

[36] Safar, M. Ageing and its effects on the cardiovascular system. *Drugs*. 1990; 39: 1-8.

[37] Smith, WM. Epidemiology of hypertension in older patients. *Am. J. Med.* 1988; 38 (Suppl. 3B): 226.

[38] Vokonas, PS; Kannel, WB; Cupples, LA. Epidemiology and risk of hypertension in the elderly: the Framingham study. *J. Hypertens*. 1988; 6 (Suppl. I): S33S9.

[39] Lonergan, ET; Krevans, MD. A national agenda for research on aging. *N. Engl. J. Med.* 1991; 324: 1825-1828.

[40] Viscoli, CM; Ostfeld, A. Epidemiology of hypertension in the elderly. In: Laragh, JH, Brenner, BM. (eds.). *Hypertension: Pathophysiology, Diagnosis, and Management*, Raven Press. New York, 1990. pp. 191-202.

[41] Strandgaard, S; Olesen, J; Skinhoj, E; Lassen, NA. Autoregulation of brain circulation in severe arterial hypertension. *Br. Med. J.* 1983; 2: 507-510.

[42] Wei, JY. Age and the cardiovascular system. *N. Engl. J. Med.* 1992; 327: 1735-1739.

[43] Marin, J; Sanchez-Ferrer, CF. Role of endothelium-formed nitric oxide on vascular responses. *Gen. Pharmacol.* 1990; 21: 575-587.

[44] Moncada, S; Palmer, RMJ; Riggs, EA. Nitric oxide: physiology, pathophysiology, and pharmacology. *Pharmacol. Rev.* 1991; 43: 109-142.

[45] Moritoki, H; Hosoki, E; Ishida, Y. Age-related decrease in endothelium-dependent dilator response to histamine in rat mesenteric artery. *Eur. J. Pharmacol.* 1986; 126: 61-67.

[46] Hynes, MR; Duckles, SP. Effect of increasing age on the endothelium-mediated relaxation of rat blood vessels in vitro. *J. Pharmacol. Exp. Therap.* 1987; 241: 387-392.

[47] Hongo, K; Nakagomi, T; Kassell, NF; Sasaki, T; Lehman, M; Vollmer, DG; Tsukahara T; Ogawa, H; Torner, J. Effects of aging and hypertension on endothelium-dependent vascular relaxation in rat carotid artery. *Stroke*. 1988; 19: 892-897.

[48] Van Brummelen, P; Buhler, FR; Kiowski, W; Amann, FW. Age-related decrease in cardiac and peripheral vascular responsiveness to isoproterenol. Studies in normal subjects. *Clin. Sci.* 1981; 60: 571-577.

[49] Gupta, M; Lipsitz, LA. Orthostatic hypotension in the elderly: diagnosis and treatment. *Am J Med.* 2007; 120: 841–847.

[50] Blacher, J; Staessen, JA; Girerd, X; Gasowski, J; Thijs, L; Wang, JG; et al. Pulse pressure not mean pressure determines cardiovascular risk in older hypertensive patients. *Arch Intern Med.* 2000; 160: 1085–1089.

[51] Luukinen, H; Koski, K; Laippala, P; Airaksinen, KE. Orthostatic hypotension and the risk of myocardial infarction in the home-dwelling elderly. *J Intern Med.* 2004; 255: 486–493.

[52] Hiitola, P; Enlund, H; Kettunen, R; Sulkava, R; Hartikainen, S. Postural changes in blood pressure and the prevalence of orthostatic hypotension among home-dwelling elderly aged 75 years or older. *Journal of Human Hypertension*. 2009; 23: 33–39.

[53] Ewing, DJ; Hume, L; Campbell, IW; Murray, A. Autonomic mechanisms in the initial heart rate response to standing. *J. Appl. Physiol.* 1980; 49: 809–814.

[54] Eagger, SA; Harvey, RJ. Clinical heterogeneity in dementia responders to cholinergic therapy. *Alzheimer Dis. Assoc. Disord.* 1995; 9 (Suppl. 2): 37–42.

[55] Guo, Z; Vintanen, M; Winblad, B; et al. Low blood pressure and incidence of dementia in a very old sample: dependent on initial cognition. *J Am Ger Soc.* 1999; 47: 723–726.

[56] De Buyzere, M; Clement, DL; Duprez, D. Chronic low blood pressure: A review. *Cardiovasc Drugs Ther.* 1998; 12: 29–35.

[57] Zhu, L; Viitanen, M; Guo, Z; et al. Blood pressure reduction, cardiovascular disease, and cognitive decline in the Mini-Mental State Examination in a community population of normal very old people: a three year follow-up. *J Clin Epidem.* 1998; 51(5): 385–391.

[58] Ruitenberg, A; Skoog, I; Ott, Am; Aevarsson, O; et al. Blood pressure and risk of dementia: results from the Rotterdam Study and the Gothenburg H-70 study. *Dementia Geriatr Cog Dis.* 2001; 12: 33–39.

[59] Brown, WD; Frackowiak; RSJ. Cerebral blood flow and metabolism studies in multi-infarct dementia. *Alzh Dis Assoc Dis.* 1991; 5:131–143.

[60] Bolster, BD; Serfaty, JM; Atalar, E. In vivo measurements of pulse wave in small vessels using intravenous MR. *Magn Reson Med.* 2001; 45:53–60.

[61] Yamamoto, Y; Akiguchi, I; Oiwa, K; et al. Adverse effect of nighttime blood pressure on the outcome of lacunar infarct patients. *Stroke.* 1998; 29: 570–576.

[62] Mehagnoul-Schipper, DJ; Colier, WN; Hoefnagels, WH; et al. Effects of furosemide versus captopril on post-prandial and orthostatic blood pressure and on cerebral oxygenation in patients _70 years old of age with heart failure. *Am J Cardiol*. 2002; 90: 596–600.
[63] Nilsson, SE; Read, S; Berg, S; et al. Low systolic blood pressure is associated with impaired cognitive function in the oldest old: longitudinal observations in a population-based sample 80 years and older. *Aging Clin Exp Res*. 2007; 19: 41–47.
[64] Faucheux, BA; Bonnet, AM; Agid, Y; Hirsch, EC. Blood vessels change in the mesencephalon of patients with Parkinson's disease. *Lancet*. 1999; 353: 981–982.
[65] Geser, F; Wenning, GK; Poewe, W; et al. How to diagnose dementia with Lewy bodies: state of the art. *Mov Disord*. 2005; 20: S11–S20.
[66] Cummings, JL; Kaufer, D. Neuropsychiatric aspects of Alzheimer's disease. The cholinergic hypothesis revisited. *Neurology*. 1996; 47: 876–883.
[67] Benarroch, EE. The central autonomic network. In: Low PA (ed) *Clinical Autonomic Disorders*. 2nd ed.New York: Lippincott-Raven, 1997; pp. 17–23.
[68] Perry, EK; Perry, RH; Blessed, G; Tomlinson, BE. A choline connection between normal aging and senile dementia in human hippocampus. *Neurosci Lett*. 1977; 6: 85-89.
[69] Whitehouse, PJ; Price, DL; Clark, AW; Coyle, JT; DeLong, MR. Alzheimer disease: evidence for selective loss of cholinergic neurons in the nucleus basalis. *Ann Neurol*. 1981; 10(2): 122-126.
[70] Perry, EK; Perry, RH; Blessed, G; Tomlinson, BE. Changes in brain cholinesterases in senile dementia of Alzheimer type. *Neuropathol Appl Neurobiol*. 1978; 4(4): 273-277.
[71] Fishman, EB; Siek, GC; MacCallum, RD; Bird, ED; Volicer, L; Marquis, JK. Distribution of the molecular forms of acetylcholinesterase in human brain: alterations in dementia of the Alzheimer type. *Ann Neurol*. 1986; 19(3): 246-252.
[72] Perry, EK; Tomlinson, BE; Blessed, G; Bergmann, K; Gibson, PH; Perry, RH. Correlation of cholinergic abnormalities with senile plaques and mental test scores in senile dementia. *BMJ*. 1978; 2 (6150): 1457-1459.

[73] Bartus, RT; Dean, RL 3rd; Beer, B; Lippa, AS. The cholinergic hypothesis of geriatric memory dysfunction. *Science*. 1982; 217(4558): 408-414.

[74] Lanctôt, KL; Herrmann, N; LouLou, MM. Correlates of response to acetylcholinesterase inhibitor therapy in Alzheimer's disease. *J Psychiatry Neurosci*. 2003; 28(1): 13-26.

[75] Jansen, RW; Lipsitz, LA. Post prandial hypotension: epidemiology, pathophysiology and clinical management. *Ann Inter Med*. 1995; 122: 286-295.

[76] Algotsson, A; Viitanen, M; Winblad, B; Solders, G. Autonomic dysfunction in Alzheimer's disease. *Acta Neuro/Scand*. 1995; 91: 14-18.

[77] Novak, P; Novak, V; Li, Z; Reimillard, G. Time-frequency analysis of slow cortical activity and cardiovascular fluctuations in a case of Alzheimer's disease. *Clin Auton Res*. 1994; 4: 141-148.

[78] Idiaquez, J; Rios, L; Sandoval, E. Postprandial hypotension in Alzheimer's disease. *Clinical Autonomic Research*. 1997; 7: 119-120.

[79] Thomaides, T; Bleasdale-Barr, K; Chaudhuri, KR; Pavitt, D; Mardsen, CD; Mathias, CJ. Cardiovascular and hormonal responses to liquid food challenge in idiopathic Parkinson's disease, multiple system atrophy, and pure autonomic failure. *Neurology*. 1993; 43: 900-904.

[80] De la Torre, JC. Is Alzheimer's disease a neurodegenerative or a vascular disorder? Data, dogma and dialectics. *Lancet Neurol*. 2004; 3: 184–190.

[81] Englund, E; Brun, A; Alling, C. White matter changes in dementia of Alzheimer's type. Biochemical and neuropathological correlates. *Brain*. 1988; 111: 1425–1439.

[82] Andin, U; Passant, U; Gustafson, L; Englund, E. Alzheimer's disease (AD) with and without white matter pathology-clinical identification of concurrent cardiovascular disorders. *Archives of Gerontology and Geriatrics*. 2007; 44: 277–286.

[83] Wang, L; Zhang, J; Xie, H. Negative relationship between severity of artherosclerosis and Alzheimer-like pathologic changes in hippocampus—a quantitative study. *Neurobiol. Aging*. 2002; 23: S490.

[84] Haglund, M; Englund, E. Cerebral amyloid angiopathy, white matter lesions and Alzheimer encephalopathy—a histopathological assessment. *Dement. Geriatr. Cogn. Disord*. 2002; 14: 161–166.

[85] Englund, E; Risberg, J; Passant, U; Gustafson, L. The appearance of white matter changes in the course of Alzheimer's disease. *Neurobiol. Aging*. 2002; 23: S489.

[86] De Leeuw, FE; Barkhof, F; Scheltens, P. Progression of cerebral white matter lesions in Alzheimer's disease: a new window for therapy? *J. Neurol. Neurosurg. Psychiatry*. 2005; 76: 1286–1288.

[87] Skoog, I. A review on blood pressure and ischaemic white matter lesions. Dement. *Geriatr. Cogn. Disord*. 1998; 9: S13–S19.

[88] Eguchi, K; Kario, K; Hoshide, S; Hoshide, Y; Ishikawa, J; Morinari, M; Hashimoto, T; Shimada, K. Greater change of orthostatic blood pressure is related to silent cerebral infarct and cardiac overload in hypertensive subjects. *Hypertens. Res*. 2004; 27: 235–241.

[89] Van Dijk, EJ; Breteler, MM; Schmidt, R; Berger, K; Nilsson, LG; Oudkerk, M; Pajak, A; Sans, S; De Ridder, M; Dufouil, C; Fuhrer, R; Giampaoli, S; Launer, LJ; Hofman, A. The association between blood pressure, hypertension, and cerebral white matter lesions: cardiovascular determinants of dementia study. *Hypertension*. 2004; 44: 625–630.

[90] Liao, D; Cooper, L; Cai, J; Toole, J; Bryan, N; Burke, G; Shahar, E; Nieto, J; Mosley, T; Heiss, G. The prevalence and severity of white matter lesions, their relationship with age, ethnicity, gender, and cardiovascular disease risk factors: the ARIC Study. *Neuroepidemiology*. 1997; 16: 149–162.

[91] De Leeuw, FE; De Groot, JC; Oudkerk, M; Witteman, JC; Hofman, A; Van Gijn, J; Breteler, MM. A follow-up study of blood pressure and cerebral white matter lesions. *Ann. Neurol*. 1999; 46: 827–833.

[92] De Leeuw, FE; Richard, F; De Groot, JC; Van Duijn, CM; Hofman, A; Van Gijn, J; Breteler, MM. Interaction between hypertension, apoE, and cerebral white matter lesions. *Stroke*. 2004; 35: 1057–1060.

[93] Dufouil, C; De Kersaint-Gilly, A; Besancon, V; Levy, C; Auffray, E; Brunnereau, L; Alperovitch, A; Tzourio, C. Longitudinal study of blood pressure and white matter hyperintensities: the EVA MRI Cohort. *Neurology*. 2001; 56: 921–926.

[94] Lazarus, R; Prettyman, R; Cherryman, G. White matter lesions on magnetic resonance imaging and their relationship with vascular risk factors in memory clinic attenders. *Int. J. Geriatr. Psychiatry*. 2005; 20: 274–279.

[95] Skoog, I; Kalaria, RN; Breteler, MM. Vascular factors and Alzheimer disease. *Alzheimer Dis. Assoc. Disord*. 1999; 13: S106–S114.

[96] Kivipelto, M; Helkala, EL; Laakso, MP; Hanninen, T; Hallikainen, M; Alhainen, K; Soininen, H; Tuomilehto, J; Nissinen, A. Midlife vascular risk factors and Alzheimer's disease in later life: longitudinal, population based study. *Br. Med. J.* 2001; 322: 1447–1451.

[97] Puisieux, F; Monaca, P; Deplanque, D; Delmaire, C; Di Pompeo, C; Monaca, C; Leys, D; Pruvo, JP; Dewailly, P. Relationship between leuko-araiosis and blood pressure variability in the elderly. *Eur. Neurol.* 2001; 46: 115–120.

[98] Burke, WJ; Coronado, PG; Schmitt, CA; Gillespie, KM; Chung, HD. Blood pressure regulation in Alzheimer's disease. *J. Auton. Nerv. Syst.* 1994; 48: 65–71.

[99] Englund, E. *A white matter disease in dementia. A study with special reference to Alzheimer's disease*. Thesis, Lund University, 1988. pp. 7–43.

[100] Erkinjuntti T. Vascular dementia: challenge of clinical diagnosis. *Int Psychogeriatr*. 1997; 9: 77–83.

[101] Pantoni, L; Rossi, R; Inzitari, D; et al. Efficacy and safety of nimodipine in subcortical vascular dementia: a subgroup analysis of the Scandinavian Multi-Infarct Dementia Trial. *J Neurol Sci*. 2000; 175: 124–134.

[102] Akiguchi, I; Tomimoto, H; Suenaga, T; et al. Alterations in glia and axons in the brains of Binswanger's disease patients. *Stroke*. 2007; 28: 1423–1429.

[103] Lishman, WA. Cerebrovascular disorders. In: Lishman, WA, Ed. *Organic Psychiatry. The Psychological Consequences of Cerebral Disorder*. 3rd ed. Oxford: Blackwell Science, 1997. pp. 375–430.

[104] Brun, A. The neuropathology of vascular dementia and its overlap with Alzheimer's Disease. In: O'Brien, J, Ames, D, Gstafson, L, et al. Eds. *Cerebrovascular disease, cognitive impairment and dementia*. London: Martin Dunitz, 2004. pp. 103–116.

[105] Englund, E. Neuropathology of white matter disease: parenchymal changes. In: Pantoni, L, Inzitari, D, Wallin, A, Eds. The Matter of White Matter. Clinical and Pathophysiological Aspects of White Matter Disease Related to Cognitive Decline and Vascular Dementia. *Current Issues in Neurodegenerative Diseases*, Vol 10. Utrecht: Academic Pharmaceutical Productions, 2000. pp. 223–246.

[106] Hebert, R; Lindsay, J; Verreault, R; et al. Vascular dementia : incidence and risk factors in the Canadian study of health and aging. *Stroke*. 2000; 31: 1487–1493.

[107] Posner, HB; Tang, MX; Luchsinger, J; et al. The relationship of hypertension in the elderly to AD, vascular dementia, and cognitive function. *Neurology*. 2002; 58: 1175–1181.

[108] Skoog, I; Gustafson, D. Hypertension and related factors in the etiology of Alzheimer Disease. *Ann NY Acad Sci*. 2002; 177: 19–36.

[109] Prince, M; Cullen, M; Mann, A. Risk factors for Alzheimer's disease and dementia: a case-control study based on the MRC elderly hypertension trial. *Neurology*. 1994; 44: 97–104.

[110] Launer, LJ; Masaki, K; Petrovitch, H; et al. The association between midlife blood pressure levels and late-life cognitive function. The Honolulu-Asia Aging Study. *JAMA*. 1995; 274: 1846–1851.

[111] Hofman, A; Ott, A; Breteler, MM; et al. Atherosclerosis, apolipoprotein E, and prevalence of dementia and Alzheimer's disease in the Rotterdam Study. *Lancet*. 1997; 349: 151–154.

[112] Forette, F; Seux, ML; Staessen, JA; et al. Prevention of dementia in randomised double-blind placebo-controlled Systolic Hypertension in Europe (Syst-Eur) trial. *Lancet*. 1998; 352(9137): 1347–1351.

[113] Qiu, C; Winblad, B; Viitanen, M; et al. Pulse pressure and risk of Alzheimer disease in persons aged 75 years and older: a communitybased, longitudinal study. *Stroke*. 2003; 34: 594–599.

[114] Mattila, K; Haavisto, M; Rajala, S; et al. Blood pressure and five years survival in the very old. BMJ. 1988; 296: 887–889.

[115] Langer, RD; Ganiato, TG; Barrett-Conner, E. Paradoxical survival of elderly men with high blood pressure. *BMJ*. 1989; 298: 1356–1358.

[116] Fletcher, AE; Bulpitt, CJ. How far should blood pressure be lowered? *N Engl J Med*. 1992; 326: 251–254.

[117] Glynn, RJ; Field, TS; Rosner, B; et al. Evidence for a positive linear relation between blood pressure and mortality in elderly people. *Lancet*. 1995; 345: 825–829.

[118] Salloway, S. Subcortical vascular dementia: Binswanger's and CADASIL. *American Academy of Neurology (AAN)* 2003; Honolulu: 8AC.006-2, 2003. pp. 1–29.

[119] Mirski, MA. Pharmacology of blood pressure management during cerebral ischemia. *American Academy of Neurology (AAN)* Miami, 2005; 5PC-004. 2005. pp. 456–469.

[120] Vasquez, J; Purve, MJ. The cholinergic pathway to cerebral blood vessels. I. Morphological studies. *Pflugers Arch*. 1979; 379: 157–163.

[121] Vanhoutte, PM. Endothelium and control of vascular function. State of the art. *Hypertension*. 1989; 13: 658–667.

[122] Wallin, A; Blennow, K; Gottfries, CG. Neurochemical abnormalities in vascular dementia. *Dementia*. 1989; 1: 120–130.

[123] Sakurada, T; Alufuzoff, I; Winblad B; et al. Substance P like immunoreactivity, choline acetyltransferase activity and cholinergic muscarinic receptors in Alzheimer's disease and multi-infarct dementia. *Brain Res*. 1990; 521(1–2): 329–332.

[124] Szilagy, AK; Nemeth, A; Martini, E; et al. Serum and CSF cholinesterase activity in various kind of dementia. *Eur Arch Psychiatry Neurol Sci*. 1987; 236: 309–311.

[125] Zaccai, J; McCracken, C; Brayne C. A systematic review of prevalence and incidence studies of dementia with Lewy bodies. *Age Ageing*. 2005; 34: 561–566.

[126] McKeith, IG; Galasko, D; Kosaka, K; et al. Consensus guidelines for the clinical and pathologic diagnosis of dementia with Lewy bodies (DLB): report of the consortium on DLB international workshop. *Neurology*. 1996; 47: 1113–1124.

[127] McKeith, IG; Perry, EK; Perry, RH. Report of the second dementia with Lewy body international workshop: diagnosis and treatment. Consortium on Dementia with Lewy Bodies. *Neurology*. 1999; 53: 902–905.

[128] McKeith, IG; Dickson, DW; Lowe, J; et al. Diagnosis and management of dementia with Lewy bodies. Third report of the DLB consortium. *Neurology*. 2005; 65: 1863–1872.

[129] Senard, JM; Rai, S; Lapeyre-Mestre, M; Brefel, C; Rascol, O; Rascol, A; Montastruc, JL. Prevalence of orthostatic hypotension in Parkinson's disease. *J Neurol Neurosurg Psychiatry*. 1997; 63: 584–589.

[130] Wenning, GK; Scherfler, C; Granata, R; Bosch, S; Verny, M; Chaudhuri, KR; Jellinger, K; Poewe, W; Litvan, I. Time course of symptomatic orthostatic hypotension and urinary incontinence in patients with postmortem confirmed parkinsonian syndromes: a clinicopathological study. *J Neurol Neurosurg Psychiatry*. 1999; 67: 620–623.

[131] Mathias, CJ; Mallipeddi, R; Bleasdale-Barr, K. Symptoms associated with orthostatic hypotension in pure autonomic failure and multiple system atrophy. *J Neurol.* 1999; 246: 893–898.
[132] Rajput, AH; Rozdilsky, B. Dysautonomia in parkinsonism: a clinicopathological study. *J Neurol Neurosurg Psychiatry.* 1976; 39: 1092–1100.
[133] Allan, LM; Ballard, CG; Allen, J; Murray, A; Davidson, AW; McKeith IG, Kenny, RA. Autonomic dysfunction in dementia. *J. Neurol. Neurosurg. Psychiatry.* 2007; 78: 671-677; originally published online 18 Dec 2006.
[134] Kaufmann, H; Nouri, S; Olanow, W; Yahr, M. Orthostatic Intolerance in Parkinson's Disease. *Neurology.* 1997; 48(suppl 2): 149.
[135] Orskov, L; Jakobsen, J; Dupont, E; de Fine Olivarius, B; Christensen, NJ. Autonomic function in Parkinsonian patients relates to duration of disease. *Neurology.* 1987; 37: 1173–1178.
[136] Thaisetthawatkul, P; Boeve, BF; Benarroch, EE; Sandroni, P; Ferman, TJ; Petersen, R; Low, PA. Autonomic dysfunction in dementia with Lewy bodies. *Neurology.* 2004; 62: 1804–1809.
[137] Peralta, C; Stampfer-Kountchev, M; Karner, E; K€ollensperger, M; Geser, F; Wolf, E; Seppi, K; Benke, T; Poewe, W; Wenning, GK. Orthostatic hypotension and attention in Parkinson's disease with and without dementia. *J Neural Transm.* 2007; 114: 585–588.
[138] Ballard, CG; Aarsland, D; McKeith, I; O'Brien, J; Gray, A; Cormack, F; Burn, D; Cassidy, T; Starfeldt, R; Larsen, JP; Brown, R; Tovee, M. Fluctuations in attention: PD dementia vs DLB with Parkinsonism. *Neurology.* 2002; 59: 1714–1720.
[139] Perlmuter, LC; Greenberg, JJ. Do you mind standing? Cognitive changes in orthostasis. *Exp Aging Res.* 1996; 22: 325–341.
[140] Ballard, C; O'Brien, J; Gray, A; Cormack, F; Ayre, G; Rowan, E; Thompson, P; Bucks, R; McKeith, I; Walker, M; Tovee, M. Attention and fluctuating attention in patients with dementia with Lewy bodies and Alzheimer disease. *Arch Neurol.* 2001; 58: 977–982.
[141] Viramo, P; Luukinen, H; Koski, K; Laippala, P; Sulkava, R; Kivela, SL. Orthostatic hypotension and cognitive decline in older people. *J Am Geriatr Soc.* 1999; 47: 600–604.
[142] Jendroska, K; Poewe, W; Daniel, SE; Pluess, J; Iwerssen-Schmidt, H; Paulsen, J; Barthel, S; Schelosky, L; Cervos-Navarro, J; DeArmond, SJ.

Ischemic stress induces deposition of amyloid beta immunoreactivity in human brain. *Acta Neuropathol (Berl)*. 1995; 90: 461–466.

[143] Graham, JG; Oppenheimer, DR. Orthostatic hypotension and nicotine sensitivity in a case of multiple system atrophy. *J Neurol Neurosurg Psychiatry*. 1969; 32: 28–34.

[144] Schrag, A; Ben-Shlomo, Y; Quinn, NP. Prevalence of progressive supranuclear palsy and multiple system atrophy: a crosssectional study. *Lancet*. 1999; 354: 1771–1775.

[145] Bower, JH; Maraganore, DM; McDonnell, SK; Rocca, WA. Incidence of progressive supranuclear palsy and multiple system atrophy in Olmsted County, Minnesota, 1976 to 1990. *Neurology*. 1997; 49: 1284–1288.

[146] Papp, MI; Kahn, JE; Lantos, PL. Glial cytoplasmic inclusions in the CNS of patients with multiple system atrophy (striatonigral degeneration, olivopontocerebellar atrophy and Shy- Drager syndrome). *J Neurol Sci*. 1989; 94: 79–100.

[147] Gilman, S; Low, P; Quinn, N; et al. Consensus statement on the diagnosis of multiple system atrophy. American Autonomic Society and American Academy of Neurology. *Clin Auton Res*. 1998; 8: 359–362.

[148] Wenning, GK; Ben Shlomo, Y; Magalhaes, M; Daniel, SE; Quinn, NP. Clinical features and natural history of multiple system atrophy. An analysis of 100 cases. *Brain*. 1994; 117: 835–845.

[149] Watanabe, H; Saito, Y; Terao, S; et al. Progression and prognosis in multiple system atrophy: an analysis of 230 Japanese patients. *Brain*. 2002; 125: 1070–1083.

[150] Den Heijer, JC; Bollen, WL; Reulen, JP; et al.. Autonomic nervous function in Huntington's disease. *Arch Neurol*. 1988; 45: 309–312.

[151] Sharma, KR; Romano, JG; Ayyar, R; Rotta, FT; Facca, A; Sanchez-Ramos, J. Sympathetic skin response and heart rate variability in patients with Huntington Disease. *Arch Neurol*. 1999; 56: 1248–1252.

[152] Andrich, J; Schmitz, T; Saft, C; et al. Autonomic nervous system function in Huntington's disease. *J Neurol Neurosurg Psychiatry*. 2002; 72: 726–731.

[153] Kobal, J; Meglicˇ, B; Mesec A; Peterlin, B. Early sympathetic hyperactivity in Huntington's disease. *European Journal of Neurology*. 2004; 11: 842–848.

[154] Mathias, CJ, Bannister, R. Dopamine _-hydroxylase de®ciency and other genetically determined causes of autonomic failure. A. Clinical

features, investigation, and management. In: *Autonomic Failure. A Textbook of Clinical Disorders of the Autonomic Nervous System*, 3rd edn (Bannister, R, Mathias, CJ. Eds). Oxford University Press, Oxford, 1992c, pp. 721-749.

[155] Heseltine, D; el-Jabri, M; Ahmed, F; Knox, J. The e€ect of ca€ein on postprandial pressure in the frail elderly. *Postgrad. Med. J.* 1991; 67: 543-547.

[156] Kunert, MP. Evaluation and management of orthostatic hypotension in elderly individuals. *J Gerontol Nurs.* 1999; 25(3): 42–46.

[157] Kaufmann, H; Brannan, T; Krakoff, L; Yahr, MD; Mandeli, J. Treatment of orthostatic hypotension due to autonomic failure with a peripheral alpha-adrenergic agonist (midodrine). *Neurology*. 1988; 38: 951–956.

[158] Wright, RA; Kaufmann, HC; Perera, R; et al. A double-blind, dose-response study of midodrine in neurogenic orthostatic hypotension. *Neurology*. 1998; 51: 120–124.

[159] Perera, R; Isola, L; Kaufmann, H. Erythropoietin improves orthostatic hypotension in primary autonomic failure. *Neurology*. 1994; 44(suppl 2): A363.

[160] Perera, R; Isola, L; Kaufmann, H. Effect of recombinant erythropoietin on anemia and orthostatic hypotension in primary autonomic failure. *Clin Auton Res.* 1995; 5: 211–213.

[161] Robertson, D; Davis, TL. Recent advances in the treatment of orthostatic hypotension. *Neurology*. 1995; 45: S26-S32.

[162] Tonkin, AL. Postural hypotension. *Med. J. Aust.* 1995; 162: 436-438.

[163] Vagaonescu, TD; Saadia, D; Tuhrim, S; Phillips, RA; Kaufmann, H. Hypertensive cardiovascular damage in patients with primary autonomic failure. *Lancet*. 2000; 355: 725–726.

[164] Maclean, AR; Allen, EV. Orthostatic hypotension and orthostatic tachycardia, treatment with the "head up" bed. *JAMA*. 1940; 115: 2162–2167.

[165] Ten Harkel, AD; Van Lieshout, JJ; Wieling, W. Treatment of orthostatic hypotension with sleeping in the head-up tilt position, alone and in combination with fludrocortisone. *J Intern Med*. 1992; 232: 139–145.

[166] Saez, T; Suarez, C; Sierra, MJ; et al. Orthostatic hypotension in the aged and its association with antihypertensive treatment. *Med Clin (Barc).* 2000; 114(14): 525–529.

[167] Masuo, K; Mikami, H ; Ogihara, T; Tuck, ML. Changes in frequency of orthostatic hypotension in elderly hypertensive patients under medications. *Am Hypertens*. 1996; 9(3): 263–268.

[168] Slavachevsky, I; Rachmani, R; Levi, Z; Brosh, D; Lidar, M; Ravid, M. Effect of enalapril and nifedipine on orthostatic hypotension in older hypertensive patients. *J Am Geriatr Soc*. 2000; 48(7): 807–810.

[169] Tinetti, ME; Baker, DI; McAvay, G; et al. A multifactorial intervention to reduce the risk of falling among elderly people living in the community. *N Engl J Med*. 1994; 331: 821–827.

[170] Lipsitz, LA; Mukai, S; Hamner, J; Gagnon, M; Babikian, V. Dynamic regulation of middle cerebral artery blood flow velocity in aging and hypertension. *Stroke*. 2000; 31: 1897–1903.

[171] Fortney, S; Tankersley, C; Lightfoot, JT; Drinkwater, D; Clulow, J; Gerstenblith, G; O'Connor, F; Becker, L; Lakatta, E; Fleg, J. Cardiovascular responses to lower body negative pressure in trained and untrained older men. *J Appl Physiol*. 1992; 73: 2693–2700.

[172] Hernandez, JP; Karandikar, A; Franke, WD. Effects of age and fitness on tolerance to lower body negative pressure. *J Gerontol [A]*. 2005; 60: 782–786.

[173] Rogers RL; Meyer JS, Mortel KF. After reaching retirement age physical activity sustains cerebral perfusion and cognition. *J Am Geriatr Soc* 1990; 38: 123–128.

[174] Franke; WD, Allbee, KA; Spencer, SE. Cerebral Blood Flow Responses to Severe Orthostatic Stress in Fit and Unfit Young and Older Adults. *Gerontology*. 2006; 52: 282–289.

In: Cardiac Rehabilitaiton
Editor: J. T. Halliday, pp. 39-73
ISBN: 978-1-60741-918-1

Chapter II

Cardiac Rehabilitation in Women

Arzu Daşkapan
Başkent University Faculty of Health Sciences, Department of Physical Therapy and Rehabilitation, Ankara/ Turkey

Abstract

Cardiovascular diseases (CVD) become the leading cause of death in the worldwide over the last decades. CVD in women brings about more disadvantages compare to men; such as later onset age, existence of other diseases and co-morbid conditions accompanying to older age. Symptoms of CVD display itself differently in women than in men, misdiagnosis is common in women. Cardiac rehabilitation (CR), targets to optimize the physical, psychological, social functioning of patients and to reduce cardiovascular morbidity and mortality. Women have a significantly lower rate of referral, are less likely to enroll and drop out before completing CR programs compared with their male counterparts. This review enlightened CVD rates in women, different aspects of women's CVD, cardiac rehabilitation objectives, components, benefits, barriers and recommendations among women.

It is well known that, risk factors play role in the development and progression of CVD. Primary and secondary prevention categories of the CR are based on the development or manifestation of atherosclerotic CVD. Both prevention efforts have same strategies. They involve cardiovascular risk reduction, encourage healthy behavior and conformity with those behaviors and support an active life style in patients with high-risk profile or CVD. Female coronary patients have higher risk factors than male. At menopause, parallel to the changes in body composition, lipid measures, insulin resistance and decline in physical activity, risk factors become more serious. CR programs lessen the risks, improve exercise tolerance, reduce stress, and increase quality of life levels. Literature supports that women benefit from CR as much as men do. Realization of health benefits is dependent on attendance and compliance to basic components of CR program (exercise training, diet etc). Some barriers included noncardiac morbidity, less social support, advanced age, high prevalence of depression and family responsibilities lessen the adherence rates in women. When this gender difference in participation rates were considered, primary prevention of CVD is crucial. 2007 The American Heart Association (AHA) guideline for CVD prevention in women, recommended the determination of women's CVD risk levels as high, intermediate, lower and optimal risk. This report also advised to take measures against CVD in either women at high risk or apparently healthy women. Lifestyle interventions in new guideline comprised smoking, physical activity, rehabilitation, dietary intake, weight reduction, omega-3 fatty acids and depression. Consequently, there is a need for future research focus on not only primary/secondary prevention but also increase the compliance of women with CR programs.

Introduction

The term of cardiovascular diseases (CVD) included diseases the heart and blood vessel system usually related to atherosclerosis [1]. CVD become the leading the cause of death and disability in worldwide over the last decades [2-3]. Breast cancer was thought as greatest health concern among women [4]. But myocardial infarction (MI), stroke and related CVD are responsible for almost twice as many deaths among women than all forms of cancer combined [5]. CVD has higher death rates, more recurrent episodes and more frequent cause of hospital admission in women than in men [6]. In Europe, more women than men die in consequence of heart disease [9]. In the United States, 54% of total CVD deaths are in women and only 46% are in men [8]. Data for England shown that coronary heart disease is responsible from almost 114 000 deaths a year and one in six occurs in women [9]. Previous study shown that: the proportion of CVD deaths in Turkey increased from 20% in 1960 to 40-50 % in 1990 [10] and contrary to expectations the coronary morbidity and mortality in premenopausal Turkish women approaches that of Turkish men [11]. New Zealand Ministry of Health reported that CVD accounted for 25.4 % of male, and 21.1 % of female deaths and the burden of disease resulting from CVD is high [12]. In Australia, CVD is a major cause of morbidity in women [13]. It seems that, heart disease is a serious health problem for ***women*** in different countries on the world.

Gender Differences Related to CVD in women

2001 Institute of Medicine report indicated clearly that the need for evaluation of sex-based differences in human disease and in medical research, with translation of these differences into clinical practice [14]. There are major differences between women and men in the pathophysiology, clinical presentation, diagnostic strategies, response to therapies and adverse outcomes of CVD [15].

It is well known that, risk factors play role in the development and progression of CVD. Traditional cardiac risk factors are essentially the same for men and women, but there are important quantitative differences between two genders. Women have smaller artery dimension, different electrical properties, and different plaque composition and development [16]. The major identified risk factors for CVD in women are tobacco use, hypertension, diabetes mellitus, dyslipidemia, obesity, sedentary lifestyle, and atherogenic diet [17]. More recently identified risk factors in women include high sensitivity C-reactive protein, homocysteine, and lipoprotein (a) [18]. Men have generally less favorable cardiac risk factors than women; on the other hand, it was found that some risk factors (diabetes mellitus, hypertension, smoking, hypercholesterolemia, and obesity) were more important for CVD in female coronary patients [19-20].

Diabetes increases CVD risk as a 3-7-fold in women compared to a 2-3-fold elevation of risk in men. Diabetes negates the presumed gender-protective effect of estrogen in premenopausal women [21]. According to estimates two-thirds of all diabetic deaths are due to CVD [22].

Hypertension is more prevalent in women than in men after the age of 65. Contrary to earlier belief, women do not tolerate effects of hypertension on cardiovascular and renal system better than men do [23]. It was observed that there was a threefold increase in CVD among women with systolic blood pressure >185 mmHg as compared with women with blood pressure <135 mmHg [24].

It was indicated that smoking is the leading cause of CVD in women younger than 50 years. The prevalence of smokers is still slightly higher in men than in women, but the decline in tobacco use among women is less evident than in men [25]. The risk in young female smokers is additionally elevated by the use of oral contraceptives [26].

There is a linear relationship between low-density lipoprotein levels and risk for CVD particularly in women less than 65 years. Additionally, low high density lipoprotein levels in women over 65 years convey a greater risk than in men [6, 27].

Obesity increases the CVD risk in women and is associated with diabetes, hypertension and dyslipidemia as well as other lifestyle-related risk factors such as physical inactivity and bad diet [19, 28].

Distribution of CVD risk factors in women may vary from country to country. It was indicated that, 23.4% of women were diabetic, 60.3% were hypertensive, and 59.7% had histories of hyperlipidemia and 9.2% smoked in United States [29]. Based on the literature, compare to white women; CVD risk levels were more remarkable among black women with higher prevalence of hypertension, obesity, diabetes and stress [30]. It was reported that; Turkish women have higher blood cholesterol levels; hypertension, diabetes and body mass index than men [31]. One study which completed in Iran shown that, prevalence of hypertension and diabetes mellitus are significantly higher in Iranian women [32]. Sasaki et al. reported that the incidence of coronary events was 60% lower in Japanese women than in men. Although the correlation of serum total cholesterol and low-density lipoprotein cholesterol concentrations to coronary events was similar in Japanese men and women, the low-density lipoprotein cholesterol concentration associated with a decreased risk of coronary events was slightly higher in women. Diabetes mellitus was a stronger risk factor in Japanese women than in men [33].

Since the late 1950s, the role of potential psychosocial risk factors had been mentioned in the development of CVD. These are Type A personality (excesses of aggression, hurry and competitiveness) and more recently type D personality (inhibition of negative emotions in social situations), depression and anxiety, low socioeconomic status, lack of social support, social isolation and chronic work stress [19]. It has been proven that low socioeconomic status as defined by occupational position, income, or education is a major psychosocial risk factor in both men and women. For example, less than 8 years of education contributed to a 4-fold risk of women (compared with women with 12 and more years of education) of developing CVD over a 14-year [34].

The transition to menopause is a complex physiological process of women's life, often accompanied by the additional effects of ageing and social adjustment [35]. Also, menopause should be considered as important period for heart disease prevention in women. Mostly, CVD is not observed in premenopausal females, especially non-smokers [36]. Incidence of cardiovascular events increases most markedly after the age of 45–54 years (i.e. at the time of the menopause) [37]. After the menopause, the incidence of MI in women also increases [38].

Menopause results from reduced secretion of the ovarian hormones estrogen and progesterone [35]. Around menopause, estrogen levels decline by 80% [39]. It is known that ovarian hormones protect against CVD. In menopausal stage, loss of ovarian function is associated with adverse metabolic changes [36, 40]. Total cholesterol and low-density lipoprotein cholesterol increased; high-density lipoprotein slightly decreased [41]. Following menopause insulin sensitivity decreased with time and insulin response to a glucose challenge [42]. There is central body fat accumulation and change in body composition [43-44]. There is a reduction in fibrinolytic activity following the menopause, and no reduction or slight increase in coagulant activity and as a result tipped towards coagulation [45]. All of these changes may explain why postmenopausal women have higher CVD risk than premenopausal women.

There are biological and gender inequalities in diagnosis, treatment, prevention and rehabilitation of ischemic heart disease [46]. The prognosis is worse for women than men [47]. One study reported that the 1-year mortality after MI is higher in women than in men [48].

Compare to men, CVD is developed in later years of life in women [49]. Among women, onset age is 10 years older and first MI time is probably 20 years older than men. This probability or thought related to late onset brings about difficulties in the prevention of CVD among young or middle aged women: these women do not attach importance to this subject and postpone taking measurements against the disease [50-51]. At the same time, advanced age is associated with co-morbid illness such as diabetes mellitus, hypertension, hypercholesterolemia, peripheral vascular disease and heart failure. These factors may play role in the worse prognosis among women with heart disease [51-53]. Later onset of CVD seems like disadvantageous rather than advantageous for women.

Symptoms of CVD display itself differently in women than in men. Atypical and non-chest pain presentations are more common in women, to the extent that it has been suggested that clinical presentation and risk factor analysis are of less value in predicting CVD for women than for men [54]. For example, chest pain is the most common presenting symptom of acute MI; however women may have atypical symptoms such as back pain, burning in the chest, abdominal discomfort, nausea, shortness of breath or fatigue. Misdiagnosis is common in women [51, 55- 56]. Existence of some previous diseases, such as arthritis, peptic ulcer disease, or chronic lung disease may cause more confusion regarding to symptoms and a missed diagnosis in the event of an acute MI [57]. The quality of the chest pain or discomfort in women is usually less severe and or milder compared to men [56]. So 50% of MI's are unrecognized in women versus 33% in men [58]. More striking and worrying result is that two thirds of women who die suddenly from heart disease had no previously recognized symptoms [59]. Early symptom recognition, prompt diagnosis and immediate treatment should be given to importance in women [1].

Many women thought their symptoms as insignificant [4]. Research reported that, women may value the health and/or well-being of others in their families over themselves [60- 62]. Women are aware of delaying symptom assessment and disease treatment to accommodate family needs [61]. Mostly women are not disposed to seek medical help and to further examination for their disease, under these conditions presentation to hospital and then starting to effective treatment are delayed [51]. Studies' findings show that women arrive an hour later to the hospital on the average, progress to more severe conditions and have a greater risk of adjusted mortality at 28 days [63]. Especially young women (< 55 years) have a worse prognosis from acute MI than their male counterparts, with a greater recurrence of MI and higher mortality [64-65].

There is need an effective diagnostic strategy for women at risk because up to 40% of initial cardiac events are fatal [66]. A consensus statement on the role of non invasive testing from the Cardiac Imaging Committee, Council on Clinical Cardiology and the Cardiovascular Imaging and Intervention Committee, Council on Cardiovascular Radiology and Intervention of the AHA relates predominantly to women with an intermediate to high likelihood of CVD before testing [67]. The 2007 AHA guideline also recommended that the determination of women's CVD risk levels [68]. For both asymptomatic and symptomatic women, initial test choice is guided by classifying women into low, intermediate, or high pretest risk categories. Patients with diabetes and peripheral arterial disease are considered to be at high risk because both diabetes and peripheral arterial disease are considered CVD risk equivalents [67]. The pretest likelihood of CVD, the characteristics of the baseline electro cardiogram, and the ability to exercise, are the major determinants of the choice of noninvasive tests [69]. American College of Cardiology/American Heart Association (ACC/AHA) exercise testing guidelines, suggested that women should undergo exercise testing if they are at an intermediate pretest risk of CAD on the basis of symptoms and risk factors, have a normal resting ECG, and are capable of maximal exercise [70]. Both the diagnostic and prognostic accuracy of exercise electro cardiogram testing could be increased by inclusion of additional parameters, such as functional capacity and treadmill scores to the classic ST-segment response [69].

For women with an abnormal resting electrocardiogram, a cardiac imaging study is recommended. Pharmacologic stress testing is preferred for women who are unable to exercise to adequate intensity [69].

If resting electrocardiogram is abnormal, an imaging modality is indicated for women. It was emphasized that stress echocardiography has greater diagnostic specificity and accuracy when compared with exercise electrocardiographic testing and it is valuable both for the recognition of CVD in women with chest pain syndromes and for their risk stratification [69].

Prevalence of nonobstructive CVD and single vessel disease is high among women. This factor induces to diminish diagnostic accuracy and higher false-positive rate for noninvasive testing in women versus men [67].

Interventions of cardiac catheterization and coronary angiography were more often among men than women, but stress testing is applied more often in women. Even among the women.who underwent coronary angiography; their testing was more delayed than was the case for men [69].

One study reported that women are less likely than men to receive angioplasty or an emergency bypass [71-72]. It was reported that gender specific physiological differences may affect treatment outcomes related to myocardial revascularization procedures and they were less favorable in women than in men [73]. Coronary vessels are smaller regardless of women's body size; so they are more prone to coronary occlusion compared to men. When revascularization is performed to reestablish blood flow to occluded arteries via percutaneous coronary intervention, or coronary artery bypass graft (CABG), the luminal diameter of an artery is a strong predictor of restenosis. In most balloon angioplasty series, women experienced higher complication and mortality rates [74]. The size of coronary vessel correlates with long term graft patency and may be associated with higher perioperative mortality rates in women after CABG [75- 76]. A recent study has confirmed that female patients CABG have a higher incidence of adverse outcomes including death, which are not mitigated by careful matching with male patients [77].

Women with heart disease have greater morbidity and mortality and have lower physical and social functioning. CVD have clear negative effects on women's physical and emotional roles in the family life. It was observed that decline in energy and activity levels and difficulties related performing household activities especially requiring upper- body movement, heavy lifting or pushing in women with heart disease [78- 79]. Following these physical inabilities coping with the CVD become difficult among women, psychological well being worsens and some problems such as lower self-esteem and feelings of guilt were seen in the women [80- 83].

It has been found that social structural and psychosocial determinants of health generally tend to be more important for women's health, whereas behavioral determinants tend to be more important for men's health [84]. Further, illness and coping behaviors to a cardiac event are influenced by male and female gender roles [85]. It was established that, housekeeping facilitates increase ability of women to deal with the stress of illness [86]. When men have severe cardiac symptoms, they tend to assume less responsibility in partnership and household activities. But women with similar symptoms try to minimize the impact of their heart disease and to avoid burdening their social contacts [87]. Because of these differences in coping with heart disease between men and women; more supportive, more encouraging and more sensitive psychosocial interventions should be planned in female cardiac patients.

It should not be ignored that screening and treating depression in women with overt CVD. Depression is prevalent problem in most of patients with heart disease [88]. Studies indicated that, after a cardiac event depression is observed in 15% and 22% of patients and women are twice as likely to suffer from depression as men Major depression and depressive symptoms worsen prognosis, reduces quality of life [89- 90]. Depression is associated with some physiologic changes, including nervous system activation, cardiac rhythm disturbances, systemic and localized inflammation and hypercoagulability, which negatively influence the cardiovascular system [91]. In patients who have CHD, depression is associated with a reduction in both short- and long-term survival [89, 92-93]. Barefoot and coauthors found that depressed individuals experienced a greater risk of mortality than did nondepressed individuals [93].

Etiological and prognostic studies indicate that depression may be a cause or a consequence of CVD [19]. Depression increases risk of adverse outcome after a diagnosis of heart disease [94]. One study related to depression following MI found that, an increased frequency of depression in women, with the greatest risk being reported in younger women [95]. This finding confirmed previous studies' opinion that possibility of an association between depression and increased adverse outcomes in younger compared with older women following both MI and myocardial revascularization procedures [23, 96- 97].

Additionally depression is an important barrier to adoption healthy lifestyle behaviors in management of heart disease [94]. Also women have specific apprehensions about emotional issues during their heart disease's recovery period. It was clearly demonstrated that, women with heart disease, need encouragement from others and peer support in this process. In this mean, group sessions may allow the sharing of knowledge and experiences and emotional support between group members [3, 98- 99].

It was indicated that women experience a poorer quality of life than men one year after acute MI [100]. Women have reported lower energy levels and more functional and psychosocial problems in quality of life subscales in other study [101- 102]. Major depression and depressive symptoms worsen prognosis, reduces quality of life [89- 90]. Women specific CVD management approaches may help to increase well-being in all areas of women's life.

Aims of Cardiac Rehabilitation

Cardiac rehabilitation (CR) targets to optimize the physical, psychological, social functioning of patients and to reduce cardiovascular morbidity and mortality [103]. Purposes for achieving these goals are to help individuals to adapt to their illness, limit or reverse the disease, modify risk factors for future cardiac illness, improve return to occupational and social functioning, and reduce the risk of re-infarction or sudden death [104-106]. Internationally CR, complete in three phases: phase one, the inpatient phase;

phase two, the outpatient phase; and phase three, the maintenance phase [107]. The first phase performs in the hospital almost immediately following a MI or cardiac event. The first phase of CR comprises patient education, basic daily activities such as sitting up in bed, joint range of motion techniques, and walking. The second phase is early recovery and performs the first few weeks to months following the hospital stay. It was targeted that increase activity levels according to patient's tolerance, and start to patient education related to lifestyle changes in this phase. Aim of third phase is to give encouragement to patient to continue regular exercise habit. This phase is important for reducing the risk of additional cardiac events and associated mortality. Finally, the third phase is the maintenance that is recommended throughout the life of the patient [108]. Significant achievements have been obtained in CR. Many studies related to CR were published in the literature and cardiac rehabilitation guidelines were issued. But CR has tended to favor men [109]. Gender specific cardiac rehabilitation programs have remained somewhat limited [110]. Some guidelines mentioned women as a specific population [111- 115]. It is seen that the few gender-specific cardiac rehabilitation programs were initiated in the recent years and these programs aimed at meeting women's need and preferences more efficiently than standard cardiac rehabilitation programs. Although existing gender-specific programs are similar to standard programs, they have women-specific goals which included positive self-concepts, assertiveness and the modification of unfavorable communication strategies [110].

Components of Cardiac Rehabilitation

Risk factor modification may be considered as milestone of CR for both prevention and management of CVD in healthy or ill individuals. 2007 American Heart Association (AHA) guideline for CVD prevention in women recommended the determination of women's CVD risk levels as high, intermediate, lower and optimal risk. Classification was done according to clinical criteria and/or the Framingham global risk score. Women who have coronary heart disease, cerebrovascular disease, peripheral arterial disease, chronic renal disease, abdominal aortic aneurysm, diabetes mellitus, and >20% of 10-year Framingham global risk takes place in high risk group. Women who have ≥1 major risk factors for CVD including cigarette smoking, poor diet, physical inactivity, obesity, family history of premature CVD, hypertension, dyslipidemia; evidence of subclinical vascular disease, metabolic syndrome, poor exercise capacity on treadmill test and/or abnormal heart rate recovery after stopping exercise takes place in risk group. Women who have <10% of Framingham global risk and a healthy lifestyle, with no risk factors takes place in optimal risk group [68]. Diabetes, dyslipidaemia, hypertension, smoking, obesity, sedentary lifestyle and poor nutrition are modifiable risk factors [68].

Primary and secondary prevention categories of the CR are based on the development or manifestation of atherosclerotic CVD. The new guideline also touches on the primary and secondary prevention of atherosclerotic vascular diseases. Both prevention efforts have same strategies. They involve cardiovascular risk reduction, encourage healthy behavior and conformity with those behaviors and support an active life style in patients with high-risk profile or CVD [55, 116].

The AHA 2007 guideline addresses issues related to lifestyle, risks to watch or avoid, and drugs to prevent heart disease. Lifestyle recommendations include leaving smoking, encouraging women to regular physical activity, adherence to healthy eating pattern, weight maintenance/ reduction, use of omega-3 fatty acids. Major risk factor interventions are maintaining optimal blood pressure, lipid and lipoprotein levels and controlling diabetes mellitus. Preventive drug interventions are aspirin therapy, beta blockers, angiotensin converting enzyme inhibitor or angiotensin receptor blocker and aldosterone blockade [68, 117].

Regular exercise is necessary component of healthy life style. Higher levels of exercise reduce both coronary risk factors (such as hypertension, obesity, diabetes) and risks of coronary heart disease [118]. It was reported that, women who are sedentary are twice as likely to develop CVD compared to women who are not sedentary [119]. But, more than 60 % of adult women fail to exercise to realize the health benefits [120]. Although physical inactivity and poor nutrition are two of most important modifiable risk factors for CVD in women, there are limited interventional studies for reducing these factors in women [121- 122]. Health-care providers should consider incentive programs which included different exercise alternatives important in women. Many women may benefit from short counseling sessions during routine office visits whereas others may need a more individualized exercise approaches. Assist and support of clinician is very helpful and useful for transition into a more active and healthier lifestyle in women [1].

CVD prevention and control strategies which directed to population are more effective than individual strategies for achieve CR targets in women [68]. Pazoki and co-workers' study shown that a community-based study can be effective for the short term adoption of physical activity behavior among women [122]. Community-based CR programs should be increased and their outcomes should be assessed.

Benefits of Cardiac Rehabilitation

When primary prevention efforts of CR for women were investigated; it is obvious that exercise have beneficial effects on CVD risk factors. Regular exercise improves blood lipid profile; leads to reduction in total cholesterol, in LDL-C and increase in HDL-C [123- 124]. Positive lipid effects of exercise may more prominent in postmenopausal women than premenopausal women [123]. Additionally regular physical activity increase exercise capacity, reduce angina symptoms and improve prognosis in cardiac patients [125-126]. It was demonstrated that; in postmenopausal women, moderate regular exercise reduced total mortality by 24-38% [127-128]. Exercise training helps to weight loss and the development of a more favorable body composition and fat distribution with regard to CVD risk [129]. Research shown that, physically active women have a more favorable waist-hip ratio than do sedentary women [130-131]. One lifestyle modification study which carried out in Turkey, shown that reduced hypertension and obesity ratio among women after training [132]. Studies shown that, regular physical activity is inversely associated with long-term cardiovascular mortality in both women and men [133- 135]. A study included postmenopausal women found that inverse relationship between leisure physical activity and cardiovascular mortality [127]. The success of the primary prevention programs for women may increase by determining the personal, psychological, and behavioral variables. After a regular participation in the prevention program, women transfer their knowledge about heart healthy behaviors to family members and/or other community members [136].

CR improves exercise tolerance, coronary risk factors, psychological well-being, and health-related quality of life in patients with heart disease [137-140]. Improvements regarding psychological well being included decreased levels of anxiety and depression, increase self esteem, and better emotional and spiritual recovery [141].

Studies suggest that secondary prevention programs of CR also reduced long-term mortality [137- 140, 142]. One trial reported that mortality reduced by 20-25% after CR programs and these gains are similar in magnitude to those of major cardiac drugs and surgery [143]. The Cochrane Database on Exercise-Based Rehabilitation for Coronary Heart Disease concluded that exercise based cardiac rehabilitation effectively reduced cardiac death, without clear evidence as to whether an exercise-only or a comprehensive cardiac rehabilitation program was more beneficial. It was found that 27% reduction in total mortality after exercise only-based rehabilitation but 13% reduction after comprehensive cardiac rehabilitation [144]. Evidence-based benefits of CR were summarized as; an improvement in exercise tolerance, improvement in symptoms, improvement in blood lipid levels, reduction in cigarette smoking, improvement in psychosocial well-being, reduction of stress, and reduction in mortality, recurrent MI, and requirement for myocardial revascularization procedures [126, 145].

Do women benefit from CR programs which devoted to secondary prevention as much as men do? The answer to this question is controversial because of there are limited data regarding exercise as secondary prevention in women. A recent systematic review and meta-analysis of randomized trials of exercise both alone and as a component of multidisciplinary CR involved women as one fifth of the cohort and included a substantial representation of both patients > 65 years of age and those following myocardial revascularization procedures[126]. An early study by Oldridge and Bitner expressed that women and men may benefit equally from CR, with improvements in clinical, psychosocial, and behavioral outcomes [146- 147]. Ades and coworkers study found that similar increase in peak aerobic capacity between males and females patients who enrolled CR program after MI and CABG [148]. Various studies on the gender-specific effectiveness of exercise exercise-based cardiac rehabilitation corroborated that women, achieved the same improvement in medical risk factors, functional capacity and quality of life [53, 102, 108, 149- 152].

On the other hand, some results were not consistent with mentioned studies reports. Two studies included women with coronary artery disease, showed no major effect on lipid values after CR [53, 108]. Allen examined risk factor management in women post CABG in his study. Results of the study demonstrated that 1 year later 58% remained obese, 54% continued to be hypertensive, and 92% continued to have elevated low-density lipoprotein cholesterol levels. These women sustained high risk profile [153]. Claesson and co workers manifested men have benefited much more than women from CR. In their study, the chance of long term survival after a myocardial infarction doubled in men during a 10 year period from the mid-1980s, whereas no improvement at all was observed in women [142]. In another CR study, compare to women, men show greater improvements in some physical components, such as body mass index [102].

Realization of health benefits is dependent on attendance and compliance to basic components of CR program (exercise training, diet etc) Robiner pointed out that, continued attention to maximizing adherence is important for enhancing treatment benefits [155]. Making instructions to subjects simpler and less demanding, addressing cognitive-motivational factors such as self-efficacy and health beliefs, offering social support and reinforcement, and providing reminders are some of developed strategies to promote adherence. Studies suggested that highest success rates are achieved by a combination of such approaches [156- 157].

Understanding patients' causal attributions regarding coronary heart disease is another important issue in terms of gains of prevention programs. Previous studies have found that attendance rates for CR or lifestyle modification programs in patients who attribute their CVD to factors apparently outside their controls, such as heredity and stress, were low [158-159].

Some studies suggested that the pattern of external attribution is more common among women than men [160- 162]. It has been speculated that this difference may be a factor responsible for low attendance by women at CR programs [162]. Education for women with heart disease should also include accurate knowledge in the area of causal attributions and beliefs about their illness.

Barriers of Cardiac Rehabilitation

Women typically have lower exercise capacity and lower exercise tolerance then men [163]. Parallel to these characteristics, some studies exhibited that, after a cardiac event it is difficult to motivate women than men to engage in regular physical activities [164- 165]. In the literature it was emphasized that women have a significantly lower rate of referral, are less likely to enroll and drop out before completing CR programs compared with their male counterparts. According to data: in the United States and Canada only approximately 25-31% of eligible patients do participate in CR programs, the rate for women being much lower at 11-20% of those eligible [166]. Similarly, different reports suggested that low levels of participation in women [167- 169].

Some barriers included advanced age, non-cardiac morbidity (such as diabetes, arthritis, and osteoporosis), high prevalence of depression and anxiety, less social support, inconvenient timings, and family responsibilities lessen the adherence rates in women [89, 147- 148, 170- 172].

Age is most consistent predictor of attendance to CR, with least attendance in younger (<49 years of age) and older (>70 years of age) women [148, 164, 173- 174]. Some researchers shown that, younger age was an independent predictor of drop out but others reported that, odds of completion doubled in patients less than 65 years of age [175- 177]. Older women often suffer from co-morbid conditions such as arthritis, osteoporosis and urinary incontinence which lessen their motivation to physical activities [178- 179]. Also it has been reported that mobility problems and difficulties in using public transportation may limit the participation in outpatient, supervised, hospital-based CR of older individuals for whom home-based CR might be a valid alternative [163, 180]. At the same time, older women do not accustomed to exercise at high intensity level and this affects negatively their participation and adherence to CR programs [181]. When planning CR programs for elderly women; age specific exercise limitations should be ruled out.

Depression makes adherence difficult to recommended behavior and lifestyle [182- 184]. It reduces the chances of successful modifications of other cardiac risk factors and participation in cardiac rehabilitation and exercise programs [183- 184]. Providing encouragement, follow-up contacts and family or partner's support may help to resolve adherence problems in depressive patients [185].

Women have more domestic tasks than men and generally women are primary caregiver for children [186- 188]. Because of general belief that caregiving is "women's work", also women undertake to caregiving of elderly and/or ill person in the family [189]. It was stated that caregivers are less likely to have time to engage in self-care and preventive health behavior than woman who do not provide care [190]. As it is well known, today most of women are professionally active [191-192]. When work related tasks were added to family responsibilities; more problems arise especially among white collar women [193- 195]. Unfortunately, female patients may give priority to domestic and work related duties, at the expense of own health. Based on observations from previous studies; women thought that attending CR would take time away from their partners, families, and friends and they were unable to attend these programs [189, 196].

Family encouragement for participation in CR is important to both men and women but encouragement from adult children is more important for women [147]. Women who do not get sufficient support from their families may refrain from become more physically active into practice [197].

Race, education, socioeconomic status, and marital status are other demographic characteristics which affect compliance with CR. Lack of insurance and lower income limit to enrollment [163, 198]. Previous studies found that there was a positive relationship between high education level and high attendance rate among women [147, 199- 202]. Apple and co-workers reported that, women have low socio-economic status and educational level enter into difficulty a lifestyle modification program which consisted of balanced and optimal nutrition, physical exercise and healthy living [203]. It was shown that as distinct from men, being married does not increase attendance at cardiac rehabilitation in women [126].

Environmental factors are important for identifying barriers to enrollment CR. They included accessibility of the program, practice norms and referral processes, and program attributes and services [204]. It was stated that geographical distance is common barrier to accessibility of CR programs for American women. When the location of CR center is too far from their home, attendance rates dropped off [163- 164, 205 -207]. Similarly, lack of transport was a problem for attending CR [196, 208]. It was found that healthcare professionals' encouragements and cardiac surgical team' refers are effective for regular attendance to CR programs in women [164, 208-210]. Consistent and encouraging feedback from CR program staff regarding progress is important to women [80, 211- 212]. Also, previous studies suggested that another important point is harmony among the program attributes and women's preferences for improving the attendance. When the program did not coordinate to their specific needs and expectations, women refused the CR programs [196]. It was observed that women's levels of self efficacy with relation to exercise and tolerance levels for physical activity were lower than men's. So women do not want to do exercise at fatigue or pain level [213-214]. Analogously, women do not prefer the predominant-male, gym-like atmosphere and the limited exercise options offered in most programs (treadmill and exercise bicycle) [212].

When considered their multidimensional barriers to CR, women oriented programs should be varied, in this sense type of program, atmosphere and exercise options should be planned according to the preferences of women. For example, home based CR programs may be good alternative especially for older, too busy women and women who have social restrictions [215- 217].

Future Suggestions

Important position of women in the family and society is unchallenged literality. Second dramatic literality is: CVD continue to threaten the life in women. There is a need to develop effective interventions for increasing achievement and popularity of CR programs for women. It should be recognized that, flexibility of CR programs is more important for women than men. When research and studies about this issue are conducted; different physiological and clinical dimensions of women's CVD, women specific psychological features, familial and social roles, needs, beliefs and expectations should be considered. It should be remembered that to protect women from heart disease is an important step for achieving a productive aging society.

References

[1] Banks, AD. Women and heart disease: missed opportunities. *J Midwifery Womens Health,* 2008, 53, 430-439.

[2] Starmba-Badiale, M; Fox, KM; Priori, SG; et al. Cardiovascular disease in women: a statement from the policy conference of the European Society of Cardiology. *Eur Heart J,* 2006, 27, 994-1005.

[3] Perry, CK; Rosenfeld, AG. Learning through connections with others: women's cardiac symptoms. *Patient Educ Couns,* 2005, 57(1), 143-146.

[4] Mosca, L; Ferris, A; Fabunmi, R; et al. Tracking women's awareness of heart disease: An American Heart Association national study. *Circulation,* 2004, 109, 573-579.

[5] American Heart Association Web site. Facts about women and cardiovascular diseases. Available at: www.americanheart.org/ presenter.jhtml?identifier=2876 *Accessed August*, 2006, 8.

[6] Bello, N; Mosca, L. Epidemiology of coronary heart disease in women. *Prog Cardiovasc Dis.,* 2004, 46, 287-295.

[7] Petersen, S; Peto, V; Rayner, M; Leal, J; Luengo-Fernandez, R; Gray, A. European cardiovascular disease statistics. 2005 edition. Oxford: British Hearth Foundation, 2005. www.heartstats.org/uploads/ documents%5 CPDF.pdf (accessed 15 Aug 2005)

[8] National Institutes of Health, National Heart, Lung and Blood Institute. Heart disease deaths in American women decline. February 1, 2007. http: //www.nih.gov/news/pr/feb2007/nhlbi-01.htm. *Accessed July*, 2007, 18.

[9] Petersen, S; Peto, V; Scarborough, P; Rayner, M. British Heart Foundation Health Promotion Research Group. Coronary heart disease statistics 2005. Oxford: *British Hearth Foundation*, 2005. www.heartstats.org/ temp/CHD_2005_Whole_spdocument.pdf (accessed 15 Aug 2005)

[10] Yalçın, M; Bardak, M. Health Statistics 1996. Republic of Turkey Ministry of Health, Research Planning and Coordination Committee. *Ankara*, 1970.

[11] Onat, A; Dursunoğlu, D; Sansoy, V. Relatively high coronary death and event rates in Turkish women; Relation to three major risk factors in five year follow-up cohort. *Int J Cardiol,* 1997, 61, 69-77.

[12] New Zealand Health Information Statistics. 2003, 7th May 2003. Mortality statistics: Totals for 1998 and 1999, (Website) New Zealand Health Information Services. Available: http://www.nzhis.govt.nz/stats/ mortstats.html [2004, 12.5.04]

[13] Australian Institute of Health and Welfare. Australian Institute of Health and Welfare National Mortality Database. Department of Health and Human Services. Canberra, Australia: Australian Institute of Health and Welfare. 1999.

[14] Wizemann, TM; Pardue, ML; (Eds); Committee on Understanding the Biology of Sex and Gender Differences, Board on Health Sciences Policy, *Institute of Medicine*, (2001) Exploring the Biological Contributions to Human Health. Does Sex Matter? Washington: National Academy Press.

[15] Wenger, NK. You've come a long way, baby: cardiovascular health disease in women: problems and prospects. *Circulation,* 2004, 109, 558-560.

[16] Legato, MJ. Gender-specific physiology: how real is it? How important is it? *Int J Fertil,* 1997, 42, 19- 29.

[17] Mosca, L; Manson, JE; Sutherland, SE; et al: Cardiovascular disease in women: A statement for healthcare professionals from the American Heart Association Writing Group. *Circulation,* 1997, 96, 2468-2482.

[18] Mosca, L. Novel cardiovascular risk factors: Do they add value to your practice? *Am Fam Physician,* 2003, 67, 264.

[19] Möller-Leihmkühler AM. Women with coronary artery disease and depression: A neglected risk group. *The World Journal of Biological Psychiatry*, 2008, 9(2), 92-101.

[20] Ades, P; Tischler, MD; Savage, PD; et al. Determinants of disability in older coronary patients. *Circulation* 1996; 94 (Suppl 1), (I-497).

[21] Eastwood, JA; Doering, LV. Gender differences in coronary artery disease. *J Cardiovasc Nurs,* 2005, 20, 340-351.

[22] Bello, N; Mosca, L. Epidemiology of coronary heart disease in women. *Prog Cardiovasc Dis,* 2004, 46, 287- 295.

[23] Vaccarino, V; Parsons, L; Every, NR; et al. Sex-based differences in early mortality after myocardial infarction. *New Engl J Med,* 1999, 41,217- 225.

[24] Van der Giezen, AM; Schopman-Geurts van Kessel, JG; Schouten, EG; et al. Systolic blood pressure and cardiovascular mortality among 13,740 Dutch women. *Prev Med*, 1990, 19, 456-465.

[25] Executive Summary. Women and smoking: A report of the Surgeon General. Morbid *Mortal Wkly Rep,* 2002, 51, 1-30

[26] Castelli, WP. Cardiovascular disease: pathogenesis, epidemiology, and risk among users of oral contraceptives who smoke. *Am J Obstet Gynecol,* 1999, 180, 349- 356

[27] Polk, ND; Naqvi, TZ. Cardiovascular disease in women: sex differences in presentation, risk factors, and evaluation. *Curr Cardiol Rep,* 2005, 7, 166-172.

[28] Kenachaiah, S; Gaziano, JM; Vasan, RS. Impact of obesity on the risk of heart failure and survival after the onset of heart failure. *Med Clin North Am,* 2004, 88, 1273-1294.

[29] Thomas, RJ; Houston Miller, N; Lamendola, C; et al. National survey on gender differences in cardiac rehabilitation programs. *J Cardiopulm Rehabil.,* 1996, 16, 402-412.

[30] Cannistra, LB; O'Malley, CJ; Balady, GJ. Comparison of outcome of cardiac rehabilitation in black women and white women. *Am J Cardiol,* 1995, 75, 890-893.

[31] Onat, A; Şurdum –Avcı, G; Şenocak, M; et al. Screening of Heart Diseases and Risk Factors Frequency in Turkey. Third Prevalence of Heart Diseases. *Turkish Cardiology Association Archive,* 1991, 19, 26-33. (Turkish).

[32] Kazemy, T; Sharifzadeh, GR. Sex differences in acute myocardial infarction in Birjand Eastern Iran. *ARYA Journal,* 2007, 3(1), 42-44.

[33] Sasaki, J; Kita, T; Mabuchi, H; et al. Gender difference in coronary events in relation to risk factors in Japanese hypercholesterolemic patients treated with low-dose simvastatin. *Circ J,* 2006, 70, 810-814.

[34] Eaker, ED. Psychosocial factors in the epidmiology of coronary heart disease in women. *Psychiatr Clin North Am,* 1989, 12, 167-173.

[35] Nelson HD. Menopause. *Lancet* 2008; 371, 760–770.

[36] Stevenson, JC. HRT and cardiovascular disease. *Best Practice & Research Clinical Obstetrics and Gynaecology,* 2009, 23, 109-120.

[37] Unal, B; Critchley, JA; Capewell, S. Explaining the decline in coronary heart disease mortality in England and Wales between 1981 and 2000. *Circulation,* 2004, 109, 1101-1107.

[38] Bugiardini, R; Bairey Merz, CN. Angina with ''normal'' coronary arteries: a changing philosophy. *JAMA,* 2005, 293, 477-84.

[39] Colditz, GA; Willett, WC; Stampfer, MJ; et al Menopause and the risk of coronary heart disease in women. *N Engl J* Med, 1987, 316,1105–1110.

[40] Kok, HS; van Asselt, KM; van der Schouv, YT; et al. Heart disease risk determines menopausal age rather than the reverse. *J Am Coll Cardiol,* 2006, 47, 1976-1983.

[41] Stevenson, JC; Crook, D; Godsland, IF. Influence of age and menopause on serum lipids and lipoproteins in healthy women. Atherosclerosis 1993, 98, 83-90.

[42] Proudler, AJ; Felton, CV; Stevenson, JC. Ageing and the response of plasma insulin, glucose and C-peptide concentrations to intravenous glucose in postmenopausal women. *Clin Sci,* 1992, 83, 489-494.

[43] Ley, CJ; Lees, B; Stevenson, JC. Sex and menopause-associated changes in body-fat distribution. *Am J Clin Nutr,* 1992, 55, 950-954.

[44] Poehlman, ET; Toth, MJ; Gardner, AW. Changes in energy balance and body composition at menopause: A controlled, longitudinal study. *Ann Intern Med,* 1995, 123, 673-675.

[45] Winkler UH. Menopause, hormone replacement therapy and cardiovascular disease: a review of haemostaseological findings. Fibrinolysis 1992; 6(Suppl 3), 5-10.

[46] Cruz, I; Serna, C; Real, J. Ischemic heart disease and primary care: identifying gender-related differences. An observational study. *BMC Family Practice,* 2008, 9, 60 doi:10.1186/1471-2296-9-60.

[47] Perry, CK; Rosenfeld, AG. Learning through connections with others: women's cardiac symptoms. *Patient Educ Couns,* 2005, 57(1), 143-146.

[48] Simon, T; Mary-Krause, M; Cambou, JP, et al.; USIC Investigators. Impact of age and gender on in-hospital and late mortality after acute myocardial infarction: increased early risk in younger women: results from the French nation-wide USIC registries. *Eur Heart J,* 2006, 27, 1282-1288.

[49] Stramba-Badiale, M; Fox, KM; Priori, SG; et al. Cardiovascular disease in women: a statement from the policy conference of the European Society of Cardiology. *Eur Heart J,* 2006, 27, 994-1005.

[50] Wenger, NK. Coronary heart disease: The female heart is vulnerable. *Prog Cardiovasc Disease,* 2003, 46, 199-229.

[51] Mikhail GW. Coronary heart disease in women. *BMJ,* 2005, 331, 467.

[52] Tofler, GH; Stone, PH; Muller, JE. Effects of gender and race on prognosis after myocardial infarction: adverse prognosis for women, particularly black women. *J Am Coll Cardiol,* 1987, 83, 484- 491.

[53] Cannistra, LB; Balady, GJ; O'Malley, CJ; et al. Comparison of the clinical profile and outcome of women and men in cardiac rehabilitation. *Am J Cardiol,* 1992, 69, 1274-1279.

[54] Sullivan, AK; Holdright, DR; Wright, CA; et al. Chest pain in women: clinical, investigative, and prognostic features. *BMJ,* 1994, 308, 883-886.

[55] Guidelines for Cardiac Rehabilitation and Secondary Prevention Programs / American *Association of Cardiovascular and Pulmonary Rehabilitation Human Kinetics*, 1999, 139-142.

[56] McSweeney, JC; Marisue, C; O'Sullivan, P; et al. Women's early warning symptoms of acute myocardial infarction. *Circulation,* 2003, 108, 2619-2123.

[57] Shephard, R; Franklin, B. Changes in the quality of life: A major goal of cardiac rehabilitation. *J Cardiopulm Rehabil,* 2001, 21, 189.

[58] Murabito, JM. Women and cardiovascular disease: Contributions from the Framingham heart study. *J Am Med Womens Assoc,* 50, 35-40, 1995.

[59] Wenger, N. Preventing cardiovascular disease in women: An update. *Clin Cardiol,* 2008, 31, 109-113.

[60] King, KM; Collins-Nakai, RL. Short term recovery from cardiac surgery in women; suggestions for practice. *Can J Cardiol,* 1998, 14, 1367-1371.

[61] King, KM; Gortner, SR. Women's short term recovery from cardiac surgery. *Prog Cardiovasc Nurs,* 1996, 11, 5-15.

[62] Meisler, JG. Toward optimal health: the experts discuss heart disease in women. *J Womens Health Gend Based MED,* 2001, 10, 17-25.

[63] Marrugat, J; Sala, J; Aboal, J. Epidemiology of cardiovascular disease. *Rev Esp Cardiol,* 2006, 59(39), 264-274.

[64] Vaccarino, V; Krumholz, HM; Yarzebski, J. Sex differences in 2-year mortality after hospital discharge for myocardial infarction. *Ann Intern Med.*, 2001, 134,173–181.

[65] Alter, DA; Naylor, CD; Austin, PC. Biology or bias: practice patterns and long-term outcomes for men and women with acute myocardial infarction, *J Am Coll Cardiol*, 2002, 39, 1909-1916.

[66] Mosca, L; Grundy, SM; Judelson, D; Guide to preventive cardiology for women: AHA/ACC Scientific Statement: consensus panel statement. *Circulation*, 1999, 99, 2480-2484.

[67] Mieres, JH; Shaw, LJ; Arai, A; et al. Role of noninvasive testing in the clinical evaluation of women with suspected coronary artery disease: consensus statement from the Cardiac Imaging Committee, Council on Clinical Cardiology, and the Cardiovascular Imaging and Intervention Committee, Council on Cardiovascular Radiology and Intervention, American Heart Association. *Circulation,* 2005, 111, 682-696.

[68] Mosca, L; Banka, CL; Benjamin, EJ; et al. Evidence Based Guidelines for Cardiovascular Disease Prevention in Women 2007 Update. *Circulation,* 2007, 115, 1481-1501.

[69] Wenger NK. Coronary heart disease in women: highlights of the past 2 years—stepping stones, milestones and obstructing boulders. *Na Clin Pract Cardıovasc Med,* 2006, 3(4), 194- 202.

[70] Gibbons, RJ; Balady, GJ; Bricker, JT; et al. American College ofCardiology/American Heart Association Task Force on Practice

Guidelines (Committee to Update the 1997 Exercise Testing Guidelines). ACC/AHA 2002 guideline update for exercise testing: summary article: a report of the American College of Cardiology/American Heart Association Task Force on Practice Guidelines (Committee to Update the 1997 Exercise Testing Guidelines). *Circulation*, 2002, 106, 1883-1892.

[71] Bellasi, A; Raggi, P; Bairey Merz, CN; et al New insights into ischemic heart disease in women. *Cleve Clin J Med,* 2007, 74(8), 585-594.

[72] Anand, SS; Xie, CC; Mehta, S; et al. Differences in the management and prognosis of women and men who suffer from acute coronary syndromes. *J Am Coll Cardiol,* 2005, 46, 1845-1851.

[73] Jacobs, AK; Johnston, JM; Haviland, A; et al. Improved outcomes for women undergoing contemporary percutaneous coronary intervention: a report from the National Heart, Lung, and Blood Institute Dynamic registry. *J Am Coll Cardiol,* 2002, 39, 1608-1614.

[74] Kelsey, SF; James, M; Holubkov, AL; et al. Results of percutaneous transluminal coronary angioplasty in women. 1985-1986 National Heart Lung and Blood Institute's Coronary Angioplasty Registry. *Circulation,* 1993, 87, 720-727.

[75] Shefier, S; Canos, M; Weinfurt, K; et al. Sex differences in coronary artery size assessed by intravascular ultrasound. *Am Heart J,* 2000, 139, 649-653.

[76] O'Connor, M; Morton, J. Effect of coronary artery diameter in patients undergoing coronary bypass surgery. *Circulation,* 1996, 93, 652-655.

[77] Kasirajan, V; Wolfe, LG; Medina, A. Institutional report – Coronary Adverse influence of female gender on outcomes after coronary bypass surgery: a propensity matched analysis. *Interactive CardioVascular and Thoracic Surgery,* 2009, 8, 408-411.

[78] Kimble, LP. Impact of cardiac symptoms on self reported household task performance in women with coronary artery disease. *J Cardiopulm Rehabil,* 2001, 21, 18-23.

[79] Wilke, NA; Sheldahl, L; Dougherty, S. Energy expenditure during household tasks in women with coronary artery disease. *Am J Cardiol,* 1995, 75, 670- 674.

[80] Moore, S; Kramer, FM. Women's views of cardiac rehabilitation programs. *J Cardiopulm Rehabil,* 1996, 16, 163-168.

[81] Charity, LA. The experiences of postmenopausal women with coronary artery disease. *West J Nurs Res.,* 1997, 19, 583-607.

[82] Charity, LA. The experiences of younger women with coronary artery disease. *J Womens Health Gend Based Med,* 1999, 8, 773-785.

[83] Hawthorne, MH. Gender differences in recovery after coronary artery surgery. *Image J Nurs Scholarsh,* 1994, 26, 75-80.

[84] Denton, M; Prus, S; Walters, V. Gender differences in health: a Canadian study of the psychosocial, structural and behavioral determinants of health. *Soc Sci Med,* 2004, 58, 2585- 2600.

[85] Lemos, K; Suls, J; Jenson, M; et al. How do female and male cardiac patients and their spouses share responsibilities after discharge from the hospital? *Ann Behav Med,* 2003, 25, 8-15.

[86] Kristofferzon, ML; Lofmark, R; Carlsson, M. Myocardial infarction: gender differences in coping and social support. *J Adv Nurs,* 2003, 44, 360-374.

[87] Mittag, O; Horres-Sieben, B; Maurischat, C. Psychological status and coping precess following ischemic heart disease: the role of age and gender. *Herzmedizin,* 2006, 23, 70-76.

[88] Ahto, M; Isoaho, R; Puolijoki, H; et al. Coronary heart disease and depression in the elderly: A population based study. *Fam Pract* 1997; 14, 436-445.

[89] Benz Scott, LA; Ben-or, K; Allen, JK. Why are women missing form outpatient cardiac rehabilitation programmes? A review of multilevel factors affecting referral, enrolment and completion. *J Womens Health,* 2002, 11, 773-791.

[90] Orth-Gomer, K. Psychosocial and behavioral aspects of cardiovascular disease prevention in men and women. *Curr Opin Psychiatry,* 2007, 20, 147-151.

[91] Miller, TQ; Smith, TW; Turner, CW; et al. A meta-analytic review of research on hostility and physical health. *Psychol Bull,* 1996, 119, 322-348.

[92] Hance, M; Carney, RM; Freedland, KE; Skala, J. Depression in patients with coronary heart disease: a 12-month follow-up. *Gen Hosp Psychiatry.,* 1996, 18, 61-65.

[93] Barefoot, JC; Helms, MJ; Mark, DB; et al. Depression and long-term mortality risk in patients with coronary artery disease. *Am J Cardiol.,* 1996, 78,613-617.

[94] Glassman, AH; O'Connor, CM; Califf, RM; et al., for the Sertraline Antidepressant Heart Attack Randomized Trial (SADHHEART) Group.

Sertraline treatment of major depression in patients with acute MI or unstable angina *JAMA,* 2002, 288, 701-709.

[95] Mallik, S; Spertus, JA; Reid, KJ; et al. Depressive Symptoms After Acute Myocardial Infarction Evidence for Highest Rates in Younger Women *Arch Intern* Med., 2006, 166, 876-883.

[96] Vaccarino, V; Abramson, JL; Emir, V; et al. Sex differences in hospital mortality alter coronary artery bypass surgery: evidence for a higher mortality in younger women. *Circulation,* 2002, 105, 1176-1181.

[97] Deshotels, A; Planchock, N; Dech, Z; et al Gender differences in perception of quality of life in cardiac rehabilitation patients. *J Cardiopulm Rehabil.,* 1995, 15(2), 143-148.

[98] Fleury, J; Sedikides, C; Lunsford, V. Women's experience following a cardiac event: the role of the self in healing. *J Cardiovasc Nurs,* 2001, 15(3), 71-82.

[99] Hagbert, V; Sjöberg, T; Ivarsson, B. Older women with a serious cardiac event experience support with a Vifladt & Hopen inspired patient group education programme. *Eur J of Cardiovasc Nurs*, 2008, 7, 140-146.

[100] Westin, L; Carlsson, R; Erhardt, L; et al. Differences in quality of life in men and women with ischemic heart disease. A prospective controlled study. *Scand Cardiovasc J,* 1999, 33(3), 160-165.

[101] Burell, G; Granlund, B. Women's hearts need special treatment. *Int J Behav Med,* 2002, 9(3), 228-242.

[102] Todaro, JF; Shen, BJ; Niaura, R. Do men and women achieve similar benefits from cardiac rehabilitation? *J Cardiopulm Rehabil,* 2004, 24(1), 45-51.

[103] Leon, AS; Franklin, BA; Costa, F; et al. Cardiac rehabilitation and secondary prevention of coronary heart disease; an American Heart Association scientific statement from the Council on Clinical Cardiology (subcommittee on exercise, cardiac rehabilitation and prevention) and the Council on Nutrition, Physical Activity and Metabolism (subcommittee on physical activity), in collaboration with the American Association of Cardiovascular and Pulmonary Rehabilitation. *Circulation,* 2005, 111, 369-376.

[104] Dinnes, J. Cardiac rehabilitation. *Nursing Times,* 1998, 94(38), 50-51.

[105] Higginson, R. Women are neglected when it comes to cardiac rehabilitation. *British Journal of Nursing,* 2003, 12(12), 713.

[106] Mitchell, R; Muggli, M; Sato, A. Cardiac rehabilitation: participating in an exercise programs in a quest to survive. *Rehabilitation Nursing,* 1999, 24(6), 236-270.

[107] Parks, D; Allison, M; Doughty Ret al. An audit of phase II cardiac rehabilitation at Auckland hospital. *New Zealand Medical Journal,* 2000, 113, 158-161.

[108] Lavie, C; Milani, R. Effects of cardiac rehabilitation and exercise training on exercise capacity, coronary risk factors, behavioral characteristics, and quality of life in women. *Am J of Cardio.* Feb, 1995, 75, 340-343.

[109] Fridlund, B. Self-related health in women after their first myocardial infarction: A 12 month comparison between participation and nonparticipation in a cardiac rehabilitation programme. *Health Care for Women International*, 2000, 21, 727-738.

[110] Bjarnason-Wehrens, B; Grande, G; Loewel, H; et al.Gender-specific issues in cardiac rehabilitation: do women with ischemic heart disease need specially tailored programmes? *Eur J Cardiovasc Prev Rehabil.,* 2007, 14, 163-171.

[111] New Zealand Guideliness Group (NZGG) and New Zealand Heart Foundation. Best practice evidence-based guidelines– cardiac rehabilitation 2002. Available at: http://www.nzgg.org.nz/guideliness/0001/Summary_resource_kit.pdf. Accessed: 25 August 2006.

[112] Stone, JA; Arthur, HM. Canadian guidelines for cardiac rehabilitation and cardiovascular disease prevention, 2nd ed. 2004: Executive summary. *Can J Cardiol,* 2005, 21(suppl D):3D-19D.

[113] American Association of Cardiovascular and Pulmonary Rehabilitation. Guidelines for cardiac rehabilitation and secondary prevention programs. Champaign: *Human Kinetics,* 2005.

[114] Wenger, NK; Froelicher, ES; Smith, LK; et al. Cardiac rehabilitation as secondary prevention. Agency for Health Care Policy and Research and National Heart, Lung and Blood Institute. *Clin Pract Guidel Quick Ref Guide Clin,* 1995, 17, 1-23.

[115] Scottish Guidelines Intercollegiate Network (SIGN). Cardiac rehabilitation. A national clinical guideline. SIGN publication no. 57. Edinburgh: SIGN; 2002.

[116] Balady, GJ; Williams, MA; Ades, PA; et al. Core components of cardiac rehabilitation/secondary prevention programs: 2007 update. A scientific statement from the American Heart Association Exercise, Cardiac

Rehabilitation, and Prevention Committee, the Council on Clinical Cardiology; the Councils on Cardiovascular Nursing, Epidemiology and Prevention, and Nutrition, Physical Activity, and Metabolism; and the American Association of Cardiovascular and Pulmonary Rehabilitation. *Circulation,* 2007, 115, 2675-82.

[117] Burrowes, JD Preventing heart disease in women. *Nutrition Today,* 2007, 42(6), 242- 247.

[118] U.S. Department of Health and Human Services: Physical activity and health: A report of Surgeon General. In Atlanta, GA: Centers of Disease Control and Prevention, National Center for Chronic Disease Prevention and Health Promotion, 1996.

[119] Centers for Disease Control and Prevention Web site, Physical activity and health. U.S. Department of Health and Human Services. Available at: www.cdc.gov/nccdphp/sgr/women. htm (Accessed April 24, 2008)

[120] U.S. Department of Health and Human Services. *Healthy People*, 2010: Understanding and improving health. Washington, DC: U.S. Government Printing Office; 2000.

[121] Koffman, DM; Bazzare, T; Mosca, L; et al. An evaluation of Choose to Move 1999; an American Heart Association physical activity program for women. *Arch Intern Med,* 2001, 161, 2193-2199.

[122] Pazoki, R; Nabipour, I; Seyednezami, N; et al. Effects of a community-based heart program on increasing healthy women's physical activity: a randomized controlled trial guided by Community-based Participatory Research (CBPR) BMC *Public Health,* 2007, 7, 216 doi: 10.1186/1471-2458-7-216.

[123] Durstine, JL; Haskell, WL. Effects of exercise training on plasma lipid and lipoproteins. *Exerc Sport Sci Rev,* 1994, 22, 477-521.

[124] Williams, PT. High-density lipoprotein cholesterol and other risk factors for coronary heart disease in female runners. *N Eng J Med,* 1996, 334; 1298-1303.

[125] Stewart, KJ; Turner, KL; Bacher, AC; et al. Are fitness, activity, and fatness associated with health-related quality of life and mood in older persons? *J of Cardiopulm Rehabil,* 2003, 23(2), 115-21.

[126] Taylor, RS; Brown, A; Ebrahim, S; et. al. Exercise-based rehabilitation for patients with coronary heart disease: systematic review and meta analysis of randomized controlled trials. *Am J Med,* 2004, 116, 682-692.

[127] Kushi, LH; Fee, RM; Folsom, AR; et al Physical activity and mortality in postmenopausal women. *JAMA,* 1997, 277, 1287-1292.

[128] Rockhill, B; Willett, WC; Manson, JE; et al. Physical activity and mortality: a prospective study among women. *Am J Public Health,* 2001, 91, 578-583.

[129] Wood, PD; Stefanick, ML; Williams, PT; et al. The effects of on plasma lipoproteins of a prudent weight-reducing diet, with or without exercise, in overweight men and women. *N Eng J Med,* 1991, 325, 461-466.

[130] Troisi, RJ; Heinhold, JW; Vokonas, PS; et al. Cigarette smoking, dietary intake, and physical activity: Effects on body fat distribution- The Normative Aging Study. *Am J Clin Nutr*, 1991, 11, 1250-1257.

[131] Wing, RR; Matthews, KA; Kuller, LH; et al. Waist to hip ratio in middle aged women. Associations with behavioral and psychosocial factors and what changes in cardiovascular risk factors. *Arterioscler Thromb,* 1991, 11, 1250-1257.

[132] Kisioglu, AN; Aslan, B; Ozturk, M; et al. Improving control of high blood pressure among middle-aged Turkish women of low socioeconomic status through public health training. *Croatian Medical Journal,* 2004, 45(4), 477-482.

[133] Paffenbarger, RS; Hyde, RT; Wing, A; et al. Physical activity, all-cause mortality, and longevity of college of alumni. *N Eng J Med,* 1986, 314, 605-613.

[134] Manson, JE; Stampfer, MJ; Colditz, GA; et al. A prospective study of exercise and incidence of myocardial infarction in women. *Circulation,* 1993, 88, 1-220.

[135] Leon, A; Connett, J; Jacobs, DR; et al. Leisure time physical activity levels and risk of coronary heart disease and death.. The Multiple Risk Factor Intervention Trial. *JAMA,* 1987, 258, 2388-2395.

[136] Halm, M; Denker, J. Primary prevention programs to reduce heart disease risk in women. *Clinical Nurse Specialist,* 2003, 17(2), 101-109.

[137] Oldridge, NB, Guyatt, GH; Fischer, ME; et al. Cardiac rehabilitation after myocardial infarction: combined experience of randomized clinical trials. *JAMA.*, 1988, 260, 945–950.

[138] O'Connor, GT; Buring, JE; Yusuf, S; et al. An overview of randomized trials of rehabilitation with exercise after myocardial infarction. *Circulation.,* 1989, 80,234–244.

[139] Williams, MA; Ades, PA; Hamm, LF; et al. Clinical evidence for a health benefit from cardiac rehabilitation: an update. *Am Heart J.,* 2006, 152, 835-8 41.

[140] Naughton, J; Dorn, J; Imamura, D. Outcomes measurement in cardiac rehabilitation: The national exercise and heart disease project. *Journal of Rehabilitation and Outcomes Measurement,* 2000, 4(4), 64-75.

[141] Conn, VS; Taylor, SG; Casey, B. Cardiac rehabilitation program participation and outcomes after myocardial infarction. *Rehabil Nurs* 1992, 17(2)58-63.

[142] Claesson, M; Burell, G; Birgander, LS; et all.. Psychosocial distress and impaired quality of life – targets neglected in the secondary prevention in women with ischemic heart disease. *Eur J Cardiovasc Prevention Rehab,* 2003, 10, 258-266.

[143] Lau, J; Antman, EM; Jimenez-Silva, et al. Cumulative meta analysis of therapeutic trials for myocardial infarction. *N Eng J Med,* 2002, 327, 248-254.

[144] Jolliffe, JA; Rees, K; Taylor, RS; et al. Exercise based rehabilitation for coronary heart disease. *Cochrane Database Syst Rev*, 2001, 1, CD001800

[145] Clark, AM; Hartling, L; Vandermeer, B; et al. Meta-analysis: secondary prevention programs for patients with coronary artery disease. *Ann Intern Med,* 2005, 143, 659-672.

[146] Oldridge, NB; LaSalle, D; Jones, NL. Exercise rehabilitation of female patients with coronaryheart disease. *Am Heart J,* 1980, 100, 755-757.

[147] Bittner, V; Sanderson, BK. Women in cardiac rehabilitation. *JAMWA,* 2003, 58, 227-235.

[148] Ades, P; Waldermann, M; Polk, D; et al. Referral patterns and exercise response in the rehabilitation of female coronary patients aged ≥ 62 years. *Am J of Cardiology,* 1992, 69, 1422-1425.

[149] Kennedy, MD; Haykowsky, M; Daub, B; et al. Effects of a comprehensive cardiac rehabilitation program on quality of life and exercise tolerance in vomen: a retrospective analysis. *Curr Control Trials Cardiovasc Med,* 2003, 4, 1.

[150] O'Farrel, P; Murray, J; Huston, P; LeGrand, C; Adamo, K. Sex differences in cardiac rehabilitation. *Can J Cardiol*, 2000, 16, 319-325.

[151] Verrill, D; Barton, C; Beasley, W; et al. Quality of life measures and gender comparisons in North Carolina Cardiac Rehabilitation Programs. *J Cardiopulm Rehabil,* 2001, 21, 37-46

[152] Balady, GJ; Jette, D; Scheer, J; et al. Changes in exercise capacity following cardiac rehabilitation in patients stratified according to age and gender. Results of Massachusetts Association of Cardiovascular and

Pıulmonary Rehabilitation Multicenter Database. *J Cardiopulm Rehabil,* 1996, 16, 38-46.

[153] Allen, JK. Coronary risk factors in women one year after coronary artery bypass grafting. *J Womens Health Gend Based Med.*, 1999, 8, 617-622.

[154] Bittner, V; Sanderson, B; Breland, J; et al. Referral patterns to a university based cardiac rehabilitation program. *Am J Cardiol,* 1999, 83, 234- 236.

[155] Robiner, WN. Enhancing adherence in clinical research. *Contemp Clin Trials,* 2005, 26, 59-77.

[156] Roter, DL; Hall, JA; Merisca, R; et al. Effectiveness of interventions to improve patient compliance: a meta-analysis. *Medical Care,* 1998, 36, 1138-1161.

[157] McDonald, HP; Garg, AX; Haynes, RB. Interventions to Enhance Patient Adherence to Medication Prescriptions: Scientific Review. *JAMA,* 2002, 288, 2868-2879.

[158] Cooper, A; Lioyd, G; Weinman, J; et al. Why patients do not attend cardiac rehabilitation: role of intentions and beliefs. *Heart,* 1999, 82, 234-246.

[159] Petrie, KJ; Weinman, J; Sharpe, N; et al. Role of patients' view of their illness in predicting return to work and functioning after myocardial infarction: longitudinal study. *BMJ,* 1996, 312, 1191-1194.

[160] Low KG, Thoresen CE, Pattillo JR et al. Causal attributions and coronary heart disease in women. *Psychol Rep,* 1993, 73, 627-636.

[161] Astin, F; Jones, K. Heart disease attributions of patients prior to elective percutaneous transluminal coronary angioplasty. *J Cardiovasc Nurs,* 2004, 19, 41-47.

[162] Furze, G &Lewin, B. Causal attributions for angina: results of an interview study. *Coron Health Care,* 2000, 4, 130-134.

[163] Halm, M; Penque, S; Doll, N; et al. Women and cardiac rehabilitation: Referral and compliance patterns. *J of Cardiovascular Nursing,* 1999. 13(3), 83-92.

[164] Gallagher, R; McKinley, S; Dracup, K. Predictors of women's attendance at cardiac rehabilitation programs. *Prog Cardiovasc Nurs,* 2003, 18, 121-126.

[165] Schuster, PM; Wright, C; Tomich, P. Gender differences in the outcomes of participants in home programs compared to those in structured cardiac rehabilitation programs. *Rehabil Nurs,* 1995, 20, 93-101.

[166] Jackson, L; Leclerc, J; Erskine, Y; et al. Getting the most of out cardiac rehabilitation; a review of referral and adherence predictors. *Heart,* 2005, 91, 10-14.

[167] Scott, IA; Eyeson-Annan, ML; Huxley, SL; et al.Optimizing care of acute myocardial infarction; results of a regional quality improvement project. *J Qual Clin Pract,* 2000, 20, 12-19.

[168] Parsk, D; Allison, M; Doughty, R; et al. An audit of phase II cardiac rehabilitation at Auckland hospital. *NZ Med J,* 2000, 113, 158-161.

[169] Evans, JA; Turner, SC; Bethell, HJN. Cardiac rehabilitation: are the NSF milestones achievable. *Heart,* 2002, 87 (Suppl) II: 41.

[170] Anderson, GL; Limacher, M; Assaf, AR; et al. Effects of conjugated equine estrogen in postmenopausal women with hysterectomy: the Women's Health Initative randomized controlled trial. *JAMA,* 2004, 291, 1701-1712.

[171] Rossow, JE; Prentice, RL; Manson, JE; et al. Postmenopausal hormone therapy and risk of cardiovascular disease by age and years since menopause. *JAMA,* 2007, 297, 1465-1477.

[172] Jacobs, AK. Coronary revascularization in women in 2003. Sex revisited. *Circulation,* 2003, 107, 375.

[173] Oldridge, NB; Ragowski, B; Gottlieb, M. Use of outpatient cardiac rehabilitation services. Factors associated with attendance. *J Cardiopulm Rehabil,* 1992, 12, 25-31.

[174] Daly, J; Sindone, AP; Thompson, DR; et al. Barriers to participation in and adherence to cardiac rehabilitation programs: a critical literature review. *Prog Cardiovasc Nurs,* 2002, 17, 8-17.

[175] Caulin-Glaser, T; Maciejewski, PK; Snow, R; et al. Depressive symptoms and sex affect completion rates and clinical outcomes in cardiac rehabilitation. *Prev Cardiol,* 2007, 10, 15-21.

[176] Yohannes, AM; Yalfani, A; Doherty, P; et al. Predictors of drop-out from an outpatient cardiac rehabilitation programme. *Clin Rehabil.* 2007, 21, 222- 229.

[177] Harrison, WN; Wardle, SA. Factors affecting the uptake of cardiac rehabilitation services in a rural locality. *Public Health,* 2005, 119, 1016-1022.

[178] Weiss, BD. Diagnostic evaluation of urinary incontinence in geriatric patients. *Am Family Physician,* 1998, 57, 2675-2684; 2688-2690.

[179] Nihira, MA; Henderson, N. Epidemiology of urinary incontinence in women. *Curr Womens Health Rep,* 2003, 3, 340-347.

[180] Marchionni, N; Fattirolli, F; Fumagalli, S; et al. Improved Exercise Tolerance and Quality of Life With Cardiac Rehabilitation of Older Patients After Myocardial Infarction Results of a Randomized, Controlled Trial. *Circulation*, 2003, 107, 2201-2206.

[181] Hasmen, P; Ceci, R; Backman, L. Exercise for older women: A training method and its influences on physical and cognitive performance. *Eur J Appl Physiol Occup Physiol,* 1992, 64, 460-466.

[182] Barefoot, JC; Burmmett, BH; Helms, MJ; et al. Depressive symptoms and survival of patients with coronary artery disease. *Psychosom Med,* 2000, 62, 790-795.

[183] Glazer, KM; Emery, CF; Frid, DJ; et al. Psychological predictors of adherence and outcomes among patients in cardiac rehabilitation. *J Cardiopulm Rehabil,* 2002, 22, 40-46.

[184] Ziegelstein, R; Fauerbach, J; Stevens, S; et al. Patients with depression are less likely to follow recommendations to reduce cardiac risk during recovery from a myocardial infarction. *Arch Intern Med,* 2000, 160, 1818-1823.

[185] Lichtman, JH; Bigger, JT; Blumenthal, JA; et al. Depression and Coronary Heart Disease: Recommendations for Screening, Referral, and Treatment: A Science Advisory From the American Heart Association Prevention Committee of the Council on Cardiovascular Nursing, Council on Clinical Cardiology, Council on Epidemiology and Prevention, and Interdisciplinary Council on Quality of Care and Outcomes Research: Endorsed by the American Psychiatric Association. *Circulation,* 2008, 118, 1768-1775.

[186] Le Bourdais, C; Hamel, PJ; Bernard, P. Le travail et l'ouvrage. Charge at partage des taches domestiques chez les couples quebecois. *Sociol Soc,* 1987, 19. 37-55

[187] Wright, EO; Shire, K; Hwang, SL; et al. The noneffects of class on the gender division of labor in the home: a comparative study of Sweden and the United States. *Gender Soc,* 1992, 6(2), 252-82.

[188] Biernat, M; Wortman, CB. Sharing of home responsibilities between professionally employed women and their husbands. *J Pers Soc Psychol,* 1991, 60, 844-860.

[189] Lane, D; Carroll, D; Ring, C; et al. Predictors of attendance at cardiac rehabilitation after myocardial infarction. *J Psychosomatic Res.,* 2001, 51, 497-501.

[190] Lee, S; Colditz, GA; Berkman, LF; et al. Caregiving and risk of coronary heart disease in us women. *Am J Prev Med,* 2003, 24(2), 113-119.

[191] Walters, W. The Social Context of Women's Health. *BMC Women's Health,* 2004, 4, S2

[192] Cohen, PN; Bianchi, SM. Marriage, children, and women's employment: what do we know? *Monthly Labor Review,* 1999, December: 22-31.

[193] Hall, EM. Gender, work control, and stress: a theoretical discussion and an empirical test. *Int J Health Services,* 1989, 19(4), 725-45.

[194] Laflamme, N; Brisson, C; Moisan, J; et al. Job strain and ambulatory blood pressure among female white-collar workers. *Scand J Work Environ Health,* 1998, 24, 334-343.

[195] Verlander, G. Female physicians: balancing career and family. *Academic Psychiatry,* 2004, 28, 331-336.

[196] Lieberman, L; Meana, M; Stewart, D. Cardiac rehabilitation: gender differences in factors influencing participation. *J Womens Health,* 1998, 7, 717-723.

[197] Moore, SM; Dolansky, MA; Ruland, CM; et al. Predictors of women's exercise maintenance after cardiac rehabilitation. *J Cardiopulm Rehabil,* 3003, 23, 40-49.

[198] Allen, JK; Scott, LB; Stewart, KJ; et al. Disparities in women's referral to and enrollment in outpatient cardiac rehabilitation. *J Gen Intern Med,* 2004, 19. 747-753.

[199] Evenson, KR; Rosamond, WD; Luepker, RV. Predictors of outpatients cardiac rehabilitation utilization: the Minnesota Heart Surgery Registry. *J Cardiopulm Rehabil.,* 1998, 18, 192-198.

[200] Johnson, SM; Karvonen, CA; Phelps, CL; et al. Assessment of analysis by gender in the Cochrane reviews as related to treatment of cardiovascular disease. *J Womens Health (Larchmt),* 2003, 12, 449-457.

[201] Husak, L; Krumholz, HM; Lin, ZQ; et al. Social support as a predictor of participation in cardiac rehabilitation after coronary bypass graft surgery *J Cardiopulm Rehabil.,* 2004, 24, 19-26.

[202] Caulin-Glaser, T; Blum, M; Schmeizl, R et al. Gender differences in referral to cardiac rehabilitation programs after revascularization. *J Cardiopulm Rehabil.*, 2001, 21, 24-30.

[203] Apple, LJ; Moore, TJ; Obarzanek, E; et al. A clinical trial of the effects of dietary patterns on blood pressure, DASH Collaborative Research Group, *N Engl J Med,* 1997, 336, 1117-1124.

[204] Parkosewich, JA. Cardiac rehabilitation barriers and opportunities among women with cardiovascular disease. *Cardiology In Review,* 2008, 16, 36-52.

[205] Evenson, KR; 6 Fleury, J. Barriers to outpatient cardiac rehabilitation participation and adherence. *J Cardiopulm Rehabil.,* 2000, 20, 241-246.

[206] Farley, RL; Wade, TD; Birchmore, L. Factors influencing attendance at cardiac rehabilitation among coronary heart disease patients. *Eur J Cardiovasc Nurs.,* 2003, 2, 205-212.

[207] Grace, SL; Evindar, A; Brooks, D; et al. Increasing patient initiation of cardiac rehabilitation referral in female percutaneus coronary intervention patients. *Can J Cardiovasc Nurs,* 2005, 15, 23-27.

[208] Heidi, HG; Schmelzer, M. Influences on women's participation in cardiac rehabilitation. *Rehabil Nurs,* 2004, 29, 116-121.

[209] Grace, SL; Scholey, P; Suskin, N; et al. A prospective comparison of cardiac rehabilitation enrollment following automatic vs usual referral. *J Rehabil Med,* 2007, 39, 239-245

[210] Harkness, K; Smith, KM; Taraba, L; et al. Effect of a postoperative telephone intervention on attendance at intake for cardiac rehabilitation after coronary artery bypass graft surgery. *Heart Lung,* 2005, 34, 179-186.

[211] Clark, AM; Barbour, RS; White, M; et al. Promoting participation in cardiac rehabilitation: patient choices and experiences. *J Adv Nurs,* 2004, 47, 5-14.

[212] Moore, SM. Women's views of cardiac rehabilitation programs. *J Cardiopulm Rehabil,* 1996, 16, 123-129.

[213] Cochrane, BL. Acute myocardial infarction in women. *Critical Care Clinics of North America,* 1992, 4, 279.

[214] Brown, V; Bryson, L; Byles, J; et al. Women's health Australia: Recruitment for a national longitudinal cohort study. *Women Health,* 1998, 28(1), 23-40.

[215] Filip, J; McGillen, C; Mosca, L. Patient preferences for cardiac rehabilitation and desired program elements. *J Cardiopulm Rehabil.,* 1999, 19, 339-343.

[216] Grace, SL; McDonald, J; Fishman, D; et al. Patient preferences for home based versus hospital-based cardiac rehabilitation. *J Cardiopulm Rehabil,* 2005, 25, 24-29.

[217] Wingham, J; Dalal, HM; Sweeney, KG; et al. Listening to patients: choice in cardiac rehabilitation. *Eur J Cardiovasc Nurs.,* 2006, 5, 289-294.

In: Cardiac Rehabilitaiton
Editor: J. T. Halliday, pp. 75-97
ISBN: 978-1-60741-918-1

Chapter III

Effects of Exercise on the Prevention and Rehabilitation of Diastolic Heart Failure

***Luis F. Joaquim*[1], *Jarbas S. Roriz-Filho*[2*], *Idiane Rosset*[3], *Matheus Roriz-Cruz*[4],**

[1]Department of Internal Medicine. School of Medicine of Ribeirão Preto at University of São Paulo, Brazil

[2]Division of Geriatrics. Department of Internal Medicine. School of Medicine of Ribeirão Preto at University of São Paulo-RP, Brazil

[3]Division of Gerontological Nursing. Faculty of Nursing. Brazilian Federal University of Rio Grande do Sul State, Brazil

[4]Division of Geriatric Medicine. Department of Internal Medicine. Brazilian Federal University of Rio Grande do Sul State, Brazil

Abstract

It is increasingly clear that exercise capacity is impaired not only in systolic, but also in diastolic heart failure (DHF). In DHF, the inability of heart to increase output during exercise is primarily due to the limited

* Corresponding author: Matheus Roriz-Cruz

Left Ventricular (LV) end-diastolic volume, despite a normal LV contractility and increased filling pressure. Healthy subjects performing exercise activity usually present an increase in heart rate that shortens diastolic filling, which results in an augmented LV filling rate that maintains or even increases LV stroke volume; this is accomplished by an enhancement of LV relaxation and a decrease in early-diastolic pressure. The mechanisms underlying an enhanced LV relaxation during exercise could involve both sympathetic stimulation and increased elastic recoil due to contractions to a lower volume. However, the adaptations in LV relaxation and early-diastolic pressure described above are not found when DHF patients are put on exercise. Indeed, LV relaxation may be acutely worsened and early-diastolic LV pressure may even increase in such a situation. Diastolic dysfunction is usually a consequence of aging, hypertrophy, ischemia, or a combination of them, and studies have shown that well-planed, long-term, increasing exercise training could favorably influence all of these effects. Accordingly, several studies have evaluated diastolic function in endurance-trained and power-trained (static exercise) patients. Among other mechanisms, endurance training prolongs the time for diastolic filling by inducing a relative sinus bradycardia secondary to either increased vagal tone or volume-induced baroceptor activation. In contrast, static exercise training results in an increased LV wall thickness relative to radius, similar to the changes following pressure-overload hypertrophy, but despite an increase in LV mass, none of the studies have demonstrated abnormal diastolic function after static training. However, repetitive lifting of greater than a few pounds should be avoided in DHF patients due to potential deleterious effects of isometric exercise on LV size and function. Therefore, based upon available data, aerobic, dynamic cardiac rehabilitation should be offered to patients with stable class II to III DHF who do not have advanced arrhythmias or another limitation to exercise. Clinical trials with appropriate outcome end-points, such as increased longevity, decreased symptoms, or improved QOL, are welcome in order to definitively prove the benefits of exercise training in patients with isolated DHF.

Keywords: Diastolic dysfunction, Diastolic heart failure, Cardiac rehabilitation, Exercise training.

Introduction

According to the ACC/AHA 2009 Guidelines Update for the Diagnosis and Management of Heart Failure in Adults [1], heart failure (HF) is a clinical situation resulted from any structural or functional cardiac disorder that makes the ventricle unable to either fill with or eject an adequate volume of blood into the great vessels, in such a manner that the heart can no longer satisfy the metabolizing tissue requirements. As the heart disorder progress, a spectrum of signs and/or symptoms can be apparent depending on which function is impaired; thus, a patient may complain of dyspnea and fatigue if cardiac output is compromised, or refer dyspnea and peripheral edema if pulmonary congestion occurs because of cardiac relaxation derangements alone [1], or even both if depressed cardiac output and fluid overload comes together. Regardless the clinical picture that dominates, HF is a syndrome that unconditionally brings exercise intolerance and loss of quality-of-life (QOL) to the patient [1].

In the past decades, two different subsets of HF have been proposed regarding the left ventricular functioning: HF with reduced ejection fraction (HFREF) and HF with preserved ejection fraction (HFPEF) [1-5]. Although the limit value of ejection fraction (EF) has been a matter of discordance among several studies, most of them has used an EF of <50% to consider systolic dysfunction, including the latest consensus about diagnosing HFPEF [6].

According to several authors, HFREF is also known as systolic HF, and it is mostly characterized by EF <50%, reduced stroke volume and work, and left ventricular (LV) eccentric remodeling which leads to increased LV diastolic volume and ultimately LV dilatation [3; 7-9]; when patients with HFREF become symptomatic, an increased LV diastolic pressure can be demonstrated, even though LV passive stiffness is in fact reduced [9].

On the other hand, HFPEF is characterized by a nondilated LV and/or a concentric LV hypertrophy or remodeling [10], and it is principally caused by LV diastolic dysfunction, where LV systolic performance (function and contractility) is in the normal range, while abnormalities in LV diastolic properties (delayed active relaxation and elevated passive stiffness) predominate and determine increased end-diastolic pressure [9]. When patients with LV diastolic dysfunction and normal or nearly normal EF present with symptoms of HF, the term "diastolic heart failure" (DHF) is preferred to differentiate it from other possible causes of HFPEF (constrictive pericarditis, valvular diseases), which do not share the same pathophysiological mechanisms [8; 9; 11; 12].

Regardless the type of HF, long-term prognosis of both systolic and diastolic HF is still poor [13], and although therapeutic approaches have been successfully performed in systolic HF in the past two decades, DHF awaits for more appropriate strategies [11; 14; 15].

Whether systolic or diastolic, one of the hallmarks in HF is the progressive reduction in exercise tolerance. In normal persons subjected to bicycle exercises, it is well-established that cardiac output increases in parallel with the peak oxygen consumption (VO_2) as a result of higher stroke volume and heart rate; in fact, stroke volume is considered to increase in response to Frank-Starling mechanisms in the ventricles, which may be impaired in DHF patients [16; 17]. Meanwhile, symptomatic patients with systolic HF and those with DHF show exercise intolerance probably due to exaggerated increases in end-diastolic and pulmonary wedge pressures pertained to a lower capability of the ventricle to accommodate larger end-diastolic volumes [17]; in fact, this may be explained by a delayed relaxation and an elevated stiffness, both characteristics of diastolic dysfunction. Furthermore, since DHF individuals may be limited to exercise training or even to daily-life activities, long-term physical deconditioning becomes of great relevance [1], and increased heart rate following exertion, which usually shortens cardiac diastole, may aggravate the entire clinical picture.

According to the stated above, the present chapter has the goal of reviewing the mechanisms involved in the reduced exercise tolerance found in patients with DHF, as well as of stressing recent cardiovascular prevention and rehabilitation strategies proposed to ameliorate the poor prognosis that still surrounds such a condition. We start briefly reviewing the pathophysiological mechanisms involved in DHF and associated exercise intolerance.

Diastolic Heart Failure - Definitions and Pathophysiology of Exercise Intolerance

Diastolic HF (DHF) has recently been described as the clinical picture of HF with a documented normal EF and signs of diastolic dysfunction, since other causes of HFPEF have been discharged (valvular heart disease, pericardial constriction, chronic obstructive pulmonary disease, etc...) [8; 9]. More specifically, according to the latest consensus statement published by the Heart Failure and Echocardiography Associations of the European Society of Cardiology, three requirements are needed to diagnose DHF: 1-) signs or symptoms of congestive HF; 2-) normal or mildly abnormal systolic LV function; and 3-) evidence of diastolic LV dysfunction [6; 10; 11]. In agreement to other studies [18; 19], it proposes that symptoms *per si* might be considered sufficient clinical evidence to suggest congestive HF, and also establishes a cut-off value of EF >50% for normal or mildly abnormal systolic function. Furthermore, as the European Committee recognizes that diastolic dysfunction can be associated to a progression in systolic HF, it proposes that LV end-diastolic and end-systolic volume indexes cannot exceed 97 mL/m2 and 49 mL/m2, respectively, in order to exclude significant LV dilatation [6].

Regarding diastolic dysfunction, the consensus establishes that documentation might come from either invasive (cardiac catheterization) or non-invasive (echocardiography) investigations. Invasive diagnostic procedure is considered the gold-standard strategy, since it allows the investigator to measure LV time constant of relaxation, end-diastolic pressure and stiffness by means of the LV pressure-volume curve, as well as pulmonary capillary wedge pressure [6]. However, since cardiac catheterization is not available in all Medical Centers, some echocardiographic parameters have been recently proposed and improved in order to estimate diastolic dysfunction; such parameters include isovolumic LV relaxation time (IVRT), ratio of early (E) to atrial (A) peaks of Doppler mitral valve flow velocity (E/A), deceleration time (DT) of early mitral valve flow velocity, ratio of pulmonary vein systolic and diastolic flow velocities, combined mitral valve and pulmonary vein blood flows, as well as tissue Doppler measurements like peak systolic shortening (S) and early diastolic lengthening (E) velocities [6; 20; 21].

All the aforementioned diagnostic criteria have been detailed elsewhere and are not part of the scope of this chapter [6; 21]. It is noteworthy that other complementary parameters may reinforce the diagnosis of DHF, such as concentric LV hypertrophy in the echocardiography and an elevated serum level of brain natriuretic peptide (BNP) [6; 11].

Diastolic HF represents about 50% of all HF cases and is mostly associated to elderly patients and women with a clinical record of essential hypertension, concentric LV hypertrophy, diabetes mellitus, obesity and, in a smaller proportion than systolic HF, cardiac ischemia [2; 9; 11; 12; 20; 22-25].

Thus, it should be expected that the pathophysiology of DHF might somehow be related to a myriad of structural and functional alterations that such conditions impose to the heart apparatus throughout their own clinical evolution. In fact, considering that the principal alterations seen in DHF are slowed LV relaxation and increased myocardial and LV chamber stiffness, which ultimately leads to compromised early and late diastolic filling, early studies have involved LV wall thickness due to hypertrophy, infiltrative disorders and also remodeling of the interstitial collagen in the DHF derangements [26-29].

Despite some controversies, mechanisms underlying the pathophysiology of DHF have been split up in those intrinsic to the cardiomyocytes and those within the extracellular matrix [9; 11; 30]. With respect to the intrinsic myocyte factors, abnormalities in the sarcolemmal calcium channels, mainly the sarcoplasmic reticulum calcium ATPase (SERCA), and also in the phosphorylation state of the proteins that influence SERCA function (phospholambam, camodulin, and calsequestrin) might both lead to an increased cytosolic calcium concentration during early and late diastole; thus, the remaining higher cytosolic calcium concentration could impair the ability of cardiac myocyte to relax and lengthen throughout the entire diastole [9; 11; 30; 31].

In addition, any circumstance affecting the myofilament contractile proteins and/or ATP hydrolysis, required in the calcium detachment from them, could alter the active relaxation and diastolic function [9; 11; 30; 31]. Finally, changes in the structural and functional characteristics of the cardiomyocyte cytoskeleton, principally in the titin isoforms, have been associated to a decreased myocardial recoiling force, which reduces LV active relaxation and increases LV passive stiffness [9; 30; 31]. It is noteworthy that all these intracellular mechanisms can somehow be modulated by adrenalin, endothelin and bradykinin receptors, as well as nitric oxide, prostaglandins and other neurohumoral pathways [32-34].

Regarding LV extracellular matrix, several studies have suggested that an imbalance in the collagen type I/collagen type III ratio and/or proteoglycans and basement membrane proteins (collagen type IV, laminin, fibronectin), together with other fiber properties (amount, geometry and degree of cross-linking), could be induced by the disease processes and neurohumoral activation [11; 30; 32; 35-46].

Therefore, the aforementioned cardiomyocyte derangements would affect the ability of the ventricle to be filled with blood while keeping diastolic pressures in normal ranges, characterizing diastolic dysfunction in either rest or during exercise [19], and a few studies have proposed that inhibition or even reversion of cardiac remodeling and dysfunction is possible if the disease process is adequately controlled by means of pharmacological and non-pharmacological therapeutic strategies [43; 45; 47; 48].

All at once, the mechanisms described above may somehow be involved in exercise intolerance found in patients suffering with DHF, since they may input some limitation to the increase in left ventricular diastolic filling and compromise cardiac output during physical efforts [17; 49-55]. In fact, after Packer [56] has pointed out to the compromised diastolic function as the most important determinant to exercise impairment, Kitzman et al [17] have shown that cardiopulmonary monitored DHF patients usually present with a reduction in stroke volume and cardiac index during a physical testing, and these alterations are mainly caused by a diminished end-diastolic volume index while peak EF and end-systolic volume index remain unaltered; similar results were found when these patients were submitted to progressive treadmill exercise and the peak oxygen consumption was monitored [49].

When echo-Doppler studies were performed while submitting patients to physical testing, an impaired myocardial relaxation was strongly associated to exercise intolerance [52] and also an increased oxidative stress [57]. Besides, most healthy people show tachycardia while exercising, and it is well-known that an increased heart rate progressively diminishes LV filling, even though some adaptations in the myocardium allow for acceleration in ventricular relaxation and guarantee lower levels of early-diastolic pressure, which increase exercise capacity [51]. However, as previously discussed, DHF patients present with a shift of the LV pressure-volume curve to higher levels of diastolic pressure, and this could be an important mechanism of intolerance when associated to tachycardia during exercise sessions [9; 51].

Together with alterations in cardiac muscle relaxation time and stiffness [54], studies have found that elderly patients with isolated DHF present with reduced distensibility and cardiac cycle-dependent changes in the aorta during exercise, which correlated with severe intolerance [58]. In addition, individuals with HF and diastolic dysfunction may experience inspiratory muscle weakness during exercise, which contributes to the dyspnea and tachypnea usually found in this situation [59].

Another condition that may influence exercise capacity is a documented LV contractile dyssynchrony documented in hypertensive patients with diastolic dysfunction or even DHF, which is markedly increased during physical stress [60]. Kato et al [53] have found that an increased systolic blood pressure is associated to impairment of exercise tolerance and also QOL in patients with DHF, which corroborates a previous report of reduced systemic vasodilatation and cardiac adaptations (increased heart rate and cardiac output) in such a condition [61]. Thus, it seems that not only the delayed myocardium relaxation-time and stiffness are involved in the physical symptoms experienced by DHF patients while exercising, but also extrinsic factors may play an important role, all of them being possible targets for drug therapeutic and cardiovascular rehabilitation.

Exercise Training in Heart Failure

It is well-established that, during aerobic activities, HF patients show an inadequate increase in cardiac output because of a multitude of factors, including submaximal increase in heart rate, impairment in LV contractility, increased end-diastolic volume (especially in dilated LV), reduced β-adrenergic responsiveness, deleterious vasoconstrictor activation (sympathetic nervous and renin-angiotensin systems), and blunted response of peripheral arterial vasodilation to exercise, all at once determining a lower blood perfusion in the active skeletal muscle [62]. Interestingly, since abnormalities in central hemodynamic function *per si* do not explain the exercise intolerance found in these patients, peripheral mechanisms have been proposed to play a role, such as endothelial function and ergoreflex activation [62].

Despite the earlier recommendations to avoid exercise activity in physical-limited HF patients [63; 64], several studies have found that exercise training in the congestive HF setting improves LV function and central hemodynamic responses (stroke volume and cardiac output) [65-70]. Exercise training also brings an improvement to peripheral hemodynamic adaptations, as endothelial functioning and vasodilatation [65; 71; 72], skeletal muscle metabolism [69; 73-75], autonomic nervous system modulation of the cardiovascular function [69; 75-78], and even the plasmatic levels of some inflammatory mediators like necrosis factor-α, interleukin-6 and nitric oxide [69; 79], which may lead to better functional capacity and QOL [47; 63; 64; 69; 74; 80-85].

For instance, Erbs et al have shown that individuals with moderate to advanced (class II-III) HF submitted to an aerobic endurance program presented with a markedly enhanced exercise capacity, as well as a significant reduction in cardiac size, together with a trend towards an increased cardiac output, and decreased pulmonary vascular and peripheral resistance at rest [83]; these results have been described in some degree in all studies cited above. Furthermore, all randomized trials have reported an improvement in maximal exercise capacity when considering gas exchange parameters such as increases in peak oxygen uptake (VO_2) and anaerobic threshold [82; 83; 86; 87].

Although most studies have been applied to HF with LV systolic dysfunction in both ischemic and non-ischemic cardiomyopathy, some researchers have also shown a significant improvement in diastolic function in these clinical settings as well, suggesting that benefits of exercise training might be extended to therapeutics and cardiac rehabilitation strategies used in isolated DHF patients [87; 88]. In fact, even when systolic dysfunction dominates the clinical picture, it seems that a reduced EF does not substantially impair exercise capacity [67; 72]. Conversely, the development of LV diastolic dysfunction may be the critical event for the compromised increase in stroke volume following Frank-Starling forces, which further reduces peak oxygen uptake during physical activity in HF [67]. Based upon the hypothesis of diastolic dysfunction having a pivotal role in exercise intolerance found in both systolic HF and isolated DHF, rehabilitation strategies acting on it need prompt development in order to having HF patients enjoying a better QOL. Even though the recent clinical controlled trial HF-ACTION has reported nonsignificant reduction in mortality and hospitalization index in HF patients submitted to exercise training [89], it also has corroborated the previous findings of better health-status and QOL [90].

In the past years, three different approaches have been proposed for exercise training in HF patients: aerobic endurance, resistance/strenght and a combination of both protocols. In a meta-analysis regarding all of these protocols, Haykowsky et al have found that only aerobic training was able to reverse left ventricular remodeling in clinically stable HF patients with diminished EF [48]. They suggested this benefit was due to a reduction in either vasoconstrictive neurohormones or hemodynamic loading, as well as alterations in the autonomic nervous system modulation of cardiovascular function, in accordance to several other authors [69; 75; 77; 78].

Aerobic training has also been associated to a reduction in peripheral arterial resistance and an increase in stroke volume, together with a decrease in the degree of cardiomegaly found in HF individuals with reduced EF, while plasmatic catecholamine levels were significantly attenuated, suggesting that neurohormonal reset is involved in the amelioration of cardiovascular function after exercise training in HF [68]. On the other hand, data from Haykowsky et al regarding strength exercise training were somewhat frustrating, since they did not show any improvement in LV remodeling [48]; they speculated that increased arterial pressure loading and LV wall stress, together with an impaired contractile and preload reserve could explain the negative results over stroke volume and EF in the protocol involving resistance training.

Despite some controversies regarding resistance exercise training, some studies have found benefits by applying this strategy to HF individuals [84; 91; 92]. In 2004, the German Federation for Cardiovascular Prevention and Rehabilitation has published recommendations for resistance exercise training, stressing that it could increase muscle strength and endurance, and ameliorate physical conditioning of HF patients [84]. Among several other benefits, authors have stated that resistance exercise could also result in better-controlled cardiovascular risk factors and bring a well-being status to the patient, mainly because of gain in muscular mass and physical functioning. Authors have also pointed out that increases in arterial blood pressure, considered potentially dangerous in HF, would depend upon the magnitude of the isometric component, as well as the load intensity and amount of muscle mass involved in the activity [84; 92]. Therefore, mainly due to this possible elevation n arterial pressure during strength exercise, they have recommended that only experienced therapists might be involved in such protocol, while specific criteria should be respected to include HF patients with lower risk for adverse reaction to resistance training programs [84; 92].

If adequately selected, HF patients could also experience a diminished peripheral arterial resistance, increased peripheral blood flow, and improved endothelial function, all considered additional effects of resistance training [91]. Meanwhile, a study by Conraads et al has suggested that a combination of endurance and resistance training may improve not only exercise parameters and LV end-systolic diameter, but also the circulatory levels of brain natriuretic peptide (BNP) [93], suggesting a potential improvement in prognosis.

When considering a specific exercise planning, it is well-established that not only the type of exercise needs to be considered, but also the intensity, frequency and duration of the activity must be part of the entire protocol for physical training in HF patients [63; 94]. In fact, recommendations from the American Heart Association (AHA) Committee on Exercise, Rehabilitation and Prevention reinforce that only subjects with stable chronic HF should be enrolled in exercise training programs [62]. The AHA Committee also reinforces that all activities should be monitored by experienced professionals who should apply individualized protocols with specific intensity, duration and frequency of the activities, while cardiovascular and respiratory parameters, such as arterial blood pressure, peak of oxygen uptake, and heart rate, this latter being carefully interpreted in those patients using β-blockers, were being frequently registered [1; 62]. Regardless the applied training approach, adherence of patients is guaranteed when supervised activities are proposed [95; 96].

While most of studies involving exercise training were applied to individuals with systolic HF, few data are available regarding the effects of exercising in DHF patients. As previously discussed in this chapter, DHF is a disorder associated to significant physical activity intolerance, probably because a multifactorial etiology involving intrinsic and extrinsic components of LV myocytes, which determines decreased LV diastolic compliance, associated to decreased aortic distensibility, increased systolic arterial pressure during exercise, cardiac dyssynchrony and possibly an alteration in skeletal muscle metabolism and activity [97; 98]. In fact, when DHF patients are put in exercise, they may not be able to increase cardiac output without a markedly increase in diastolic pressures because of an impaired LV relaxation, as well as a reduction in end-diastolic volume due to a shortened diastole during tachycardia [62]. Additionally, Kato et al have identified that systolic arterial pressure is markedly increased in DHF subjects during exercise, which further compromises LV relaxation and end-diastolic pressure [99]. If so, this latter result would relatively contraindicate resistance physical training in DHF, since this kind of exercise increases arterial blood pressure depending on the grade of isometric activity applied [84; 92].

As DHF is commonly associated to elderly women, hypertension, concentric LV hypertrophy, obesity, diabetes mellitus and, in a smaller proportion, myocardial ischemic disease, it is speculated that, at least in part, exercise training might improve physical capacity in DHF patients by means of interfering with these risk factors [1; 62].

Recently, an exercise protocol has been applied in old rats with documented diastolic dysfunction by means of LV pressure-volume curves and, even though experimentally, the authors have shown that training protocol partially reverted changes observed in cardiac function and remodeling caused by aging [100]. Also, it has been proved in chronic HF rats that 8-week swimming program is able to improve LV end-diastolic pressure, skeletal muscle metabolism and also plasmatic levels of the inflammatory marker interleukin-10 [101]. These results are in accordance to other experimental procedures in rats with diastolic dysfunction [102]. In view of the cardiovascular effects associated to aerobic/endurance exercise training, such as reversibility of LV remodeling, reduction of vasoconstrictive neurohumoral factors, improvement of sympathovagal balance, and relative bradycardia [48], it seems that such a protocol could have significant influence over risk factors related to DHF with potential positive impact on QOL and mortality.

Observational studies have demonstrated that well-planed, home-based, monitored exercise training in women with DHF has had a great impact in reducing symptoms and perceptions, and therefore improving QOL [103; 104]. According to the authors, women with NYHA class III DHF showed the greatest increase in distance walked on the 6-minutes walking test, which ultimately expressed in better QOL scores, and this effect seemed to be independently from pharmacological therapy [103; 104]. They also described that those women with DHF not engaged in an exercise program presented deterioration in functional performance during the period of observation. In older women with stable NYHA class II to III submitted to a 12-week, home-based, low-to-moderate-intensity combined walking and education program, a substantial improvement was noted in physical capacity, depressive symptoms, sleep pattern, and finally in QOL [105; 106], suggesting that current ongoing clinical trials with appropriate outcome end-points, such as increased longevity, decreased symptoms, or improved QOL, may definitively prove the benefits of exercise training in patients with isolated DHF.

Conclusion

Physical training has been used as an adjuvant therapy in the management of HF for the past years, and markedly improvement in cardiovascular and respiratory indexes has been associated to either endurance or resistance training protocols. Most guidelines have established that only stable HF patients should be enrolled in exercise training, and protocols should be applied and supervised by experienced therapists.

With respect to resistance training, absolute contraindications should be observed before its application to HF patients, such as unstable angina pectoris, uncontrolled arterial blood pressure and/or arrhythmias, severe valve diseases, and hypertrophic obstructive cardiomyopathy, and possibly extended to aerobic exercise strategies. Regardless of the exercise protocol chosen, most clinical trials have been evaluated physical training in systolic HF, and few results are available for DHF. Nevertheless, since endurance/aerobic exercise training seems to attenuate cardiovascular derangements in HF patients such as LV remodeling, vasoconstrictive neurohumoral input, sympathovagal imbalance, and a endothelial dysfunction, among other risk factors potentially found in DHF, some researchers have proposed its application on cardiac rehabilitation programs to DHF patients.

Conversely,, resistance training should be avoided in DHF subjects, since the increase in arterial blood pressure and heart rate observed in such protocol could have a potential deleterious effect on the reduced LV relaxation and enhanced diastolic pressures usually found in this disorder. Clinical trials with appropriate outcome end-points, such as reduced mortality and improved QOL, are needed in order to definitively establish the benefits of exercise training in patients with isolated DHF. Meanwhile, efforts must be done in order to enroll DHF patients in a complete management of risk factors, such as reducing plasmatic glucose and lipid levels, controlling blood pressure and heart rate, as well as starting regular physical activity as a strategy to prevent development of LV hypertrophy in hypertensive individuals [107].

References

[1] Hunt, SA; Abraham, WT; Chin, MH; Feldman, AM; Francis, GS; Ganiats, TG; Jessup, M; Konstam, MA; Mancini, DM; Michl, K; Oates, JA; Rahko, PS; Silver, MA; Stevenson, LW; Yancy, CW. 2009 Focused Update Incorporated Into the ACC/AHA 2005 Guidelines for the Diagnosis and Management of Heart Failure in Adults. A Report of the American College of Cardiology Foundation/American Heart Association Task Force on Practice Guidelines developed in collaboration with the International Society for Heart and Lung Transplantation. *J. Am. Coll. Cardiol.,* 2009, 53(15), e1-e90.

[2] Bursi, F; Weston, SA; Redfield, MM; Jacobsen, SJ; Pakhomov, S; Nkomo, VT; Meverden, RA; Roger VL. Systolic and diastolic heart failure in the community. *JAMA,* 2006, 296(18), 2209-2216.

[3] Chatterjee, K; Massie, B. Systolic and diastolic heart failure: differences and similarities. *J. Cardiac. Fail.,* 2007, 13(7), 569-576.

[4] European Society of Cardiology; Heart Failure Association of the ESC (HFA); European Society of Intensive Care Medicine (ESICM), Dickstein, K; Cohen-Solal, A; Filippatos, G; McMurray, JJV; Ponikowski, P; Poole-Wilson, PA; Strömberg, A; van Veldhuisen, DJ; Atar, D; Hoes, AW; Keren, A; Mebazaa, A; Nieminem, M; Priori, SG; Swedberg, K. ESC guidelines for the diagnosis and treatment of acute and chronic heart failure 2008. The Task Force for the Diagnosis and Treatment of Acute and Chronic Heart Failure 2008 of the European Society of Cardiology. *Eur. J. Heart Fail.,* 2008, 10(10), 933-989.

[5] Yamamoto, K; Sakata, Y; Ohtani, T; Takeda, Y; Mano, T. Heart failure with preserved ejection fraction - what is known and unknown. *Circ. J.,* 2009, 73(3), 404-410.

[6] Paulus, WJ; Tschöpe, C; Sanderson, JE; Rusconi, C; Flachskampf, FA; Rademakers, FE; Marino, P; Smiseth, OA; De Keulenaer, G; Leite-Moreira, AF; Borbély, A; Édes, I; Handoko, ML; Heymans, S; Pezzali, N; Pieske, B; Dickstein, K; Fraser, AG; Brutsaert, DL. How to diagnose diastolic heart failure: a consensus statement on the diagnosis of heart failure with normal left ventricular ejection fraction by the Heart Failure and Echocardiography Associations of the European Society of Cardiology. *Eur. Heart J.,* 2007, 28(20), 2539-2550.

[7] Zile, MR; Brutsaert, DL. New concepts in diastolic dysfunction and diastolic heart failure - Part I: diagnosis, prognosis, and measurements of diastolic function. *Circulation,* 2002, 105(11), 1387-1393

[8] Zile, MR. Heart failure with preserved ejection fraction: is this diastolic heart failure? *J. Am. Coll. Cardiol.,* 2003, 41(9), 1519-1522.

[9] Zile, MR; Baicu, CF; Bonnema, DD. Diastolic heart failure: definitions and terminology. *Prog. Cardiov. Dis.,* 2005, 47(5), 307-313.

[10] Maeder, MT; Kaye, DM. Heart failure with normal left ventricular ejection fraction. *J. Am. Coll. Cardiol.,* 2009, 51(11), 905-918.

[11] Ouzounian, M; Lee, DS; Liu, PP. Diastolic heart failure: mechanisms and controversies. *Nat. Clin. Pract. Cardiovasc. Med.,* 2008, 5(7), 375-386.

[12] McDonald, K. Diastolic heart failure in the elderly: underlying mechanisms and clinical relevance. *Int. J. Cardiol.,* 2008, 125(2), 197-202.

[13] Franklin, KM; Aurigemma, GP. Prognosis in diastolic heart failure. *Prog. Cardiov. Dis.,* 2005, 47(5), 333-339.

[14] Brutsaert, DL; Sys, SU; Gillebert, TC. Diastolic failure: pathophysiology and therapeutic implications. *J. Am. Coll. Cardiol.,* 1993, 22(1), 318-325.

[15] MacCarthy PA; Kearney MT; Nolan J; Lee AJ; Prescott RJ; Shah AM; Brooksby, WP; Fox, KAA. Prognosis in heart failure with preserved left ventricular systolic function: prospective cohort study. *BMJ,* 2003, 327(7406), 78-79.

[16] Higginbotham, MB; Morris, KG; Williams, RS; McHale, PA; Coleman, RE; Cobb, FR. Regulation of stroke volume during submaximal and maximal upright exercise in normal man. *Circ. Res.,* 1986, 58(2), 281-291.

[17] Kitzman, DW; Higginbotham, MB; Cobb, FR; Sheikh, KH; Sullivan, MJ. Exercise intolerance in patients with heart failure and preserved left ventricular systolic function: failure of the Frank-Starling mechanism. *J. Am. Coll. Cardiol.,* 1991, 17(5), 1065-1072.

[18] Vasan, RS; Levy, D. Defining diastolic heart failure: a call for standardized diagnostic criteria. *Circulation,* 2000, 101(17), 2118-2121.

[19] Yturralde, FR; Gaasch, WH. Diagnostic criteria for diastolic heart failure. *Prog. Cardiov. Dis.,* 2005, 47(5), 314-319.

[20] Aurigemma, GP; Gaasch, WH. Clinical practice: diastolic heart failure. *N. Engl. J. Med.* 2004, 351(11), 1097-1105.

[21] Quiñones, MA. Assessment of diastolic function. *Prog. Cardiov. Dis.,* 2005, 47(5), 340-355.

[22] Kitzman, DW; Gardin, JM; Gottdiener, JS; Arnold, A; Boineau, R; Aurigemma, G; Marino, EK; Lyles, M; Cushman, M; Enright, PL. Importance of heart failure with preserved systolic function in patients ≥65 years of age. *Am. J. Cardiol.,* 2001, 87(4), 413-419.

[23] Kitzman, DW. Diastolic heart failure in the elderly. *Heart Fail. Rev.,* 2002, 7(1), 17-27.

[24] Desai, A. Current understanding of heart failure with preserved ejection fraction. *Curr. Opin. Cardiol.,* 2007, 22(6), 578-585.

[25] Dhar, S; Koul, D; D'Alonzo Jr, GE. Current concepts in diastolic heart failure. *J. Am. Osteopath. Assoc.,* 2008, 108(4), 203-209.

[26] Bache, RJ. Effects of hypertrophy on the coronary circulation. *Prog. Cardiov. Dis.,* 1988, 30(6), 403-440.

[27] Gilbert, JC; Glantz, SA. Determinants of left ventricular filling and of the diastolic pressure-volume relation. *Circ. Res.,* 1989, 64(5), 827-852.

[28] Morgan, JP. Abnormal intracellular modulation of calcium as a major cause of cardiac contractile dysfunction. *N. Engl. J. Med.,* 1991, 325(9), 625-632.

[29] Litwin, SE; Grossman, W. Diastolic dysfunction as a cause of heart failure. *J. Am. Coll. Cardiol.,* 1993, 22 (suppl. A), 49A-55A.

[30] Zile, MR; Brutsaert, DL. New concepts in diastolic dysfunction and diastolic heart failure - Part II: causal mechanisms and treatment. *Circulation,* 2002, 105(12), 1503-1508.

[31] Borbély, A; van der Velden, J; Papp, Z; Bronzwaer, JGF; Edes, I; Stienen, GJM; Paulus, WJ. Cardiomyocyte stiffness in diastolic heart failure. *Circulation,* 2005, 111(6), 774-781.

[32] Hogg, K; McMurray, J. Neurohumoral pathways in heart failure with preserved systolic function. *Prog. Cardiov. Dis.,* 2005, 47(6), 357-366.

[33] Brutsaert, DL. Cardiac dysfunction in heart failure: the cardiologist's love affair with time. *Prog. Cardiov. Dis.,* 2006, 49(3), 157-181.

[34] Ladeiras-Lopes, R; Ferreira-Martins, J; Leite-Moreira, AF. Acute neurohumoral modulation of diastolic function. *Peptides,* 2009, 30(2), 419-425.

[35] Borg, TK; Caulfield, JB. The collagen matrix of the heart. *Fed. Proc.*, 1981, 40(7), 2037–2041.

[36] Weber, KT. Cardiac interstitium in health and disease: the fibrillar collagen network. *J. Am. Coll. Cardiol.*, 1989, 13(7), 1637–1652.

[37] Jalil, JE; Doering, CW; Janicki, JS; Pick, R; Shroff, SG; Weber, KT. Fibrillar collagen and myocardial stiffness in the intact hypertrophied rat left ventricle. *Circ. Res.*, 1989, 64(6), 1041–1050.

[38] Covell, JW. Factors influencing diastolic function: possible role of the extracellular matrix. *Circulation,* 1990, 81(suppl III), III-155–III-158.

[39] Weber, KT; Janicki, JS; Pick, R; Capasso, J; Anversa, P. Myocardial fibrosis and pathologic hypertrophy in the rat with renovascular hypertension. *Am. J. Cardiol.*, 1990, 65(14), 1G-7G.

[40] Weber, KT; Brilla, CG. Pathological hypertrophy and cardiac interstitium: fibrosis and renin-angiotensin-aldosterone system. *Circulation,* 1991, 83(6), 1849–1865.

[41] Villari, B; Campbell, SE; Hess, OM; Mall, G; Vassalli, G; Weber, KT; Krayenbuehl, HP. Influence of collagen network on left ventricular systolic and diastolic function in aortic valve disease. *J. Am. Coll. Cardiol.* 1993, 22(5), 1477-1484.

[42] Weber, KT; Sun, Y; Guarda, E. Structural remodeling in hypertensive heart disease and the role of hormones. *Hypertension,* 1994, 23(6 Pt 2), 869–877.

[43] Villari, B; Vassalli, G; Monrad, ES; Chiariello, M; Turina, M; Hess, OM. Normalization of diastolic dysfunction in aortic stenosis late after valve replacement. *Circulation,* 1995, 91(9), 2353–2358.

[44] Kato, S; Spinale, FG; Tanaka, R; et al. Inhibition of collagen cross-linking: effects on fibrillar collagen and ventricular diastolic function. *Am. J. Physiol.*, 1995, 269 (*Heart Circ. Physiol.* 38), H863–H868.

[45] Brilla, CG; Funck, RC; Rupp, H. Lisinopril-mediated regression of myocardial fibrosis in patients with hypertensive heart disease. *Circulation,* 2000, 102(12), 1388–1393.

[46] Martos, R; Baugh, J; Ledwidge, M; O'Loughlin, C; Conlon, C; Patle, A; Donnelly, SC; McDonald, K. Diastolic heart failure: evidence of increased myocardial collagen turnover linked to diastolic dysfunction. *Circulation,* 2007, 115(7), 888-895.

[47] Giannuzzi, P; Temporelli, PL; Corrà, U; Tavazzi, L. Antiremodeling effect of long-term exercise training in patients with stable chronic heart failure. Results of the Exercise in Left Ventricular Dysfunction and Chronic Heart Failure (ELVD-CHF) trial. *Circulation,* 2003, 108, 554-559.

[48] Haykowsky, MJ; Liang, Y; Pechter, D; Jones, LW; McAlister, FA; Clark, AM. A meta-analysis of the effect of exercise training on left ventricular remodeling in heart failure patients. The benefit depends on the type of training performed. *J. Am. Coll. Cardiol.,* 2007, 49(24), 2329-2336.

[49] Davies, SW; Fussel, AL; Jordan, SL; Poole-Wilson, PA; Lipkin, DP. Abnormal diastolic filling patterns in chronic heart failure - relationship to exercise capacity. *Eur. Heart J.,* 1992, 13(6), 749-757.

[50] Spiranova, L; Toman, J; Stejfa, M; Soucek, M; Richter, M; Kara, T. Systolic and diastolic function in patients with chronic heart failure at rest and during exercise. *Int. J. Cardiol.,* 1997, 59(3), 251-256.

[51] Little, WC; Kitzman, DW; Cheng, CP. Diastolic dysfunction as a cause of exercise intolerance. *Heart Fail. Rev.,* 2000, 5(4), 301-306.

[52] Rovner, A; Greenberg, NL; Thomas, JD; Garcia, MJ. Relationship of diastolic intraventricular pressure gradients and aerobic capacity in patients with diastolic heart failure. *Am. J. Physiol. Heart Circ. Physiol.,* 2005, 289(5), H2081-H2088.

[53] Kato, S; Onishi, K; Yamanaka, T; Takamura, T; Dohi, K; Yamada, N; Wada, H; Nobori, T; Ito, M. Exaggerated hypertensive response to exercise in patients with diastolic heart failure. *Hypertens. Res.,* 2008, 31(4), 679-684.

[54] Westermann, D; Kasner, M; Steendijk, P; Spillmann, F; Riad, A; Weitmann, K; Hoffmann, W; Poller, W; Pauschinger, M; Schultheiss, HP; Tschöpe, C. Role of left ventricular stiffness in heart failure with normal ejection fraction. *Circulation,* 2008, 117(16), 2051-2060.

[55] Barmeyer, A; Müllerleile, K; Mortensen, K; Meinertz, T. Diastolic dysfunction in exercise and its role for exercise capacity. *Heart Fail. Rev.,* 2009, 14(2), 125-34.

[56] Packer, M. Abnormalities of diastolic function as a potential cause of exercise intolerance in chronic heart failure. *Circulation,* 1990, 81(2 Suppl.), III78-III86.

[57] Dekleva, M; Celic, V; Kostic, N; Pencic, B; Ivanovic, AM; Caparevic, Z. Left ventricular diastolic dysfunction is related to oxidative stress and exercise capacity in hypertensive patients with preserved systolic function. *Cardiology,* 2007, 108(1), 62-70.

[58] Hundley, WG; Kitzman, DW; Morgan, TM; Hamilton, CA; Darty, SN; Stewart, KP; Herrington, DM; Link, KM; Little, WG. Cardiac cycle-dependent changes in aortic area and distensibility are reduced in older patients with isolated diastolic heart failure and correlate with exercise intolerance. *J. Am. Coll. Cardiol.,* 2001, 38(3), 796-802.

[59] Lavietes, MH; Gerula, CM; Fless, KG; Cherniack, NS; Arora, RR. Inspiratory muscle weakness in diastolic dysfunction. *Chest* 2004, 126(3), 838-844.

[60] Wang, YC; Hwang, JJ; Lai, LP; Tsai, CT; Lin, LC; Katra, R; Lin, JL. Coexistence and exercise exacerbation of intraleft ventricular contractile dyssynchrony in hypertensive patients with diastolic heart failure. *Am. Heart J.,* 2007, 154(2), 278-284.

[61] Borlaug, BA; Melenovsky, V; Russell, SD; Kessler, K; Pacak, K; Becker, LC; Kass, DA. Impaired chronotropic and vasodilator reserves limit exercise capacity in patients with heart failure and a preserved ejection fraction. *Circulation,* 2006, 114(20), 2138-2147.

[62] Piña, IL; Chair Writing Group; Apstein, CS; Balady, GJ; Belardinelli, R; Chaitman, BR; Duscha, BD; Fletcher, BJ; Fleg, JL; Myers, JN; Sullivan, MJ. Exercise and heart failure: a statement from the American Heart Association Committee on Exercise, Rehabilitation, and Prevention. *Circulation,* 2003, 107(8), 1210-1225.

[63] Wielenga, RP; Coats, AJS; Mosterd, WL; Huisveld, IA. The role of exercise training in chronic heart failure. *Heart,* 1997, 78(5), 431-436.

[64] Rubin, SA. Exercise training in heart failure - contradictory or conventional? *J. Am. Coll. Cardiol.,* 2007, 49(24), 2337--2340.

[65] Sullivan, MJ; Higginbotham, MB; Gobb, FR. Exercise training in patients with severe left ventricular dysfunction: hemodynamic and metabolic effects. *Circulation,* 1988, 78(3), 506-515.

[66] Coats, AJ; Adamopoulos, S; Meyer, TE; Conway, J; Sleight, P. Effects of physical training in chronic heart failure. *Lancet,* 1990, 335(8692), 63-66.

[67] Sullivan, MJ; Cobb, FR. Central hemodynamic response to exercise in patients with chronic heart failure. *Chest,* 1992, 101(5 Suppl.), 340S-346S.

[68] Hambrecht, R; Gielen, S; Linke, A; Fiehn, E; Yu, J; Walther, C; Schoene, N; Schuler, G. Effects of exercise training on left ventricular function and peripheral resistance in patients with chronic heart failure: a randomized trial. *JAMA,* 2000, 283(23), 3095-3101.

[69] Warburton, DE; Taylor, A; Bredin, SS; Esch, BT; Scott, JM; Haykowsky, MJ. Central haemodynamics and peripheral muscle function during exercise in patients with chronic heart failure. *Appl. Physiol. Nutr. Metab.* 2007, 32(2), 318-331.

[70] Mezzani, A; Corrà, U; Giannuzzi, P. Central adaptations to exercise training in patients with chronic heart failure. *Heart Fail. Rev.,* 2008, 13(1), 13-20.

[71] Hambrecht, R; Fiehn, E; Weigl, C; Gielen, S; Hamann, C; Kaiser, R; Yu, J; Adams, V; Niebauer, J; Schuler, G. Regular physical exercise corrects endothelial dysfunction and improves exercise capacity in patients with chronic heart failure. *Circulation,* 1998, 98(24), 2709-2715.

[72] Duscha, BD; Schulze, PC; Robbins, JL; Forman, DE. Implications of chronic heart failure on peripheral vasculature and skeletal muscle before and after exercise training. *Heart Fail. Rev.,* 2008, 13(1), 21-37.

[73] Mancini, DM; Walter, G; Reichek, N; Lenkinski, R; McCully, KK; Mullen, JL; Wilson, JR. Contribution of skeletal muscle atrophy to exercise intolerance and altered muscle metabolism in heart failure. *Circulation,* 1992, 85(4), 1364-1373.

[74] McKelvie, RS; Teo, KK; McCartney, N; Humen, D; Montague, T; Yusuf, S. Effects of exercise training in patients with congestive heart failure: a critical review. *J. Am. Coll. Cardiol.,* 1995, 25(3), 789-796.

[75] Negrao, CE; Middlekauff, HR. Adaptations in autonomic function during exercise training in heart failure. *Heart Fail. Rev.,* 2008, 13(1), 51-60.

[76] Kiilavuori, K; Toivonen, L; Näveri, H; Leinonen, H. Reversal of autonomic derangements by physical training in chronic heart failure assessed by heart rate variability. *Eur. Heart J.,* 1995, 16(4), 490-495.

[77] Radaelli, A; Coats, AJ; Leuzzi, S; Piepoli, M; Meyer, TE; Calciati, A; Finardi, G; Bernardi, L; Sleight, P. Physical training enhances sympathetic and parasympathetic control of heart rate and peripheral vessels in chronic heart failure. *Clin. Sci. (Lond.),* 1996, 91(Suppl.), 92-94.

[78] Roveda, F; Middlekauff, HR; Rondon, MU; Reis, SF; Souza, M; Nastari, L; Barreto, AC; Krieger, EM; Negrão, CE. The effects of exercise training on sympathetic neural activation in advanced heart failure: a randomized controlled trial. *J. Am. Coll. Cardiol.,* 2003, 42(5), 854-860.

[79] Niebauer, J. Effects of exercise training on inflammatory markers in patients with heart failure. *Heart Fail. Rev.,* 2008, 13(1), 39-49.

[80] Belardinelli, R; Georgiou, D; Cianci, G; Purcaro, A. Randomized, controlled trial of long-term moderate exercise training in chronic heart failure. Effects on functional capacity, quality of life, and clinical outcome. *Circulation,* 1999, 99(9), 1173-1182.

[81] European Heart Failure Training Group. Experience from controlled trials of physical training in chronic heart failure. Protocol and patient factors in effectiveness in the improvement in exercise tolerance. *Eur. Heart J.,* 1998, 19(3), 466-475.

[82] Dubach, P; Sixt, S; Myers, J. Exercise training in chronic heart failure: why, when and how. *Swiss Med Wkly,* 2001, 131(35-36), 510-514.

[83] Erbs, S; Linke, A; Gielen, S; Fiehn, E; Walther, C; Yu, J; Adams, V; Schuler, G; Hambrecht, R. Exercise training in patients with severe chronic heart failure: impact on left ventricular performance and cardiac

size. A retrospective analysis of the Leipzig Heart Failure Training Trial. *Eur. J. Cardiovasc. Prev. Rehabil.*, 2003, 10(5), 336-344.

[84] Bjarnason-Wehrens, B; Mayer-Berger, W; Meister, ER; Baum, K; Hambrecht, R; Gielen, S. Recommendations for resistance exercise in cardiac rehabilitation. Recommendations of the German Federation for Cardiovascular Prevention and Rehabilitation. *Eur. J. Cardiovasc. Prev. Rehabil.*, 2004, 11, 352-361.

[85] van Tol, BA; Huijsmans, RJ; Kroon, DW; Schothorst, M; Kwakkel, G. Effects of exercise training on cardiac performance, exercise capacity and quality of life in patients with heart failure: a meta-analysis. *Eur. J. Heart Fail.*, 2006, 8(8), 841-850.

[86] Demopoulos, L; Bijou, R; Fergus, I; Jones, M; Strom, J; LeJemtel, TH. Exercise training in patients with severe congestive heart failure: enhancing peak aerobic capacity while minimizing the increase in ventricular wall stress. *J. Am. Coll. Cardiol.*, 1997, 29(3), 597-603.

[87] Myers, J; Wagner, D; Schertler, T; Beer, M; Luchinger, R; Klein, M; Rickli, H; Muller, P; Mayer, K; Schwitter, J; Dubach, P. Effects of exercise training on left ventricular volumes and function in patients with nonischemic cardiomyopathy: application of magnetic resonance myocardial tagging. *Am. Heart J.*, 2002, 144, 719-725.

[88] Belardinelli, R; Georgiou, D; Cianci, G; Berman, N; Ginzton, L; Purcaro, A. Exercise training improves left ventricular diastolic filling in patients with dilated cardiomyopathy. Clinical and prognostic implications. *Circulation,* 1995, 91(11), 2775-2784.

[89] O'Connor, CM; Whellan, DJ; Lee, KL; Keteyian, SJ; Cooper, LS; Ellis, SJ; Leifer, ES; Kraus, WE; Kitzman, DW; Blumenthal, JA; Rendall, DS; Miller, NH; Fleg, JL; Schulman, KA; McKelvie, RS; Zannad, F; Piña, IL; HF-ACTION Investigators. Efficacy and safety of exercise training in patients with chronic heart failure: HF-ACTION randomized controlled trial. *JAMA,* 2009, 301(14), 1439-1450.

[90] Flynn, KE; Piña, IL; Whellan, DJ; Lin, L; Blumenthal, JA; Ellis, SJ; Fine, LJ; Howlett, JG; Keteyian, SJ; Kitzman, DW; Kraus, WE; Miller, NH; Schulman, KA; Spertus, JA; O'Connor, CM; Weinfurt, KP. Effects of exercise training on health status in patients with chronic heart failure: HF-ACTION randomized controlled trial. *JAMA,* 2009, 301(14), 1451-1459.

[91] Umpierre, D; Stein, R. Hemodynamic and vascular effects of resistance training: implications for cardiovascular diseases. *Arq. Bras. Cardiol.*, 2007, 89(4), 233-239.

[92] Braith, RW; Beck, DT. Resistance exercise: training adaptations and developing a safe exercise prescription. *Heart Fail. Rev.*, 2008, 13(1), 69-79.

[93] Conraads, VM; Beckers, P; Vaes, J; Martin, M; van Hoof, V; De Maeyer, C; Possemiers, N; Wuyts, FL; Vrints, CJ. Combined endurance/resistance training reduces NT-proBNP levels in patients with chronic heart failure. *Eur. Heart J.*, 2004, 25(20), 1797-1805.

[94] Wisløff, U; Støylen, A; Loennechen, JP; Bruvold, M; Rognmo, Ø; Haram, PM; Tjønna, AE; Helgerud, J; Slørdahl, SA; Lee, SJ; Videm, V; Bye, A; Smith, GL; Najjar, SM; Ellingsen, Ø; Skjærpe, T. Superior cardiovascular effect of aerobic interval training versus moderate continuous training in heart failure patients. A randomized study. *Circulation,* 2007, 115(24), 3086-3094.

[95] McKelvie, RS; Teo, KK; Roberts, R; McCartney, N; Humen, D; Montague, T; Hendrican, K; Yusuf, S. Effects of exercise training in patients with heart failure: the exercise rehabilitation trial (EXERT). *Am. Heart J.*, 2002, 144(1), 23–30.

[96] Barbour, KA; Miller, NH. Adherence to exercise training in heart failure: a review. *Heart Fail. Rev.*, 2008, 13(1), 81-89.

[97] Kitzman, DW. Exercise intolerance. *Prog. Cardiov. Dis.* 2005, 47(6), 367-379.

[98] Little, WC; Brucks, S. Therapy for diastolic heart failure. *Prog. Cardiov. Dis.*, 2005, 47(6), 380-388.

[99] Kato, S; Onishi, K; Yamanaka, T; Takamura, T; Dohi, K; Yamada, N; Wada, H; Nobori, T; Ito, M. Exaggerated hypertensive response to exercise in patients with diastolic heart failure. *Hypertens. Res.*, 2008, 31(4), 679-684.

[100] Choi, SY; Chang, HJ; Choi, S; Kim, K; Cho, YS; Youn, TJ; Chung, WY; Chae, IH; Choi, DJ; Kim, HS; Kim, CH; Oh, BH; Kim, MH. Long-term exercise training attenuates age-related diastolic dysfunction: association of myocardial collagen cross-linking. *J. Korean Med. Sci.*, 2009, 24(1), 32-39.

[101] Nunes, RB; Tonetto, M; Machado, N; Chazan, M; Heck, TG; Veiga, ABG; Dall'Ago, P. Physical exercise improves plasmatic levels of IL-

10, left ventricular end-diastolic pressure, and muscle lipid peroxidation in chronic heart failure rats. *J. Appl. Physiol.,* 2008, 104(6), 1641-1647.

[102] Brenner, DA; Apstein, CS; Saupe, KW. Exercise training attenuates age-associated diastolic dysfunction in rats. *Circulation,* 2001, 104(2), 221-226.

[103] Gary, RA; Sueta, CA; Dougherty, M; Rosenberg, B; Cheek, D; Preisser, J; Neelon, V; McMurray, R. Home-based exercise improves functional performance and quality of life in women with diastolic heart failure. *Heart Lung,* 2004, 33(4), 210-218.

[104] Gary, RA; Sueta, CA; Rosenberg, B; Cheek, D. Use of the 6-minute walk test for women with diastolic heart failure. *J. Cardiopulm. Rehabil.,* 2004, 24(4), 264-268.

[105] Gary, R. Exercise self-efficacy in older women with diastolic heart failure: results of a walking program and education intervention. *J. Gerontol. Nurs.,* 2006, 32(7), 31-39.

[106] Gary, R; Lee, SY. Physical function and quality of life in older women with diastolic heart failure: effects of a progressive walking program on sleep patterns. *Prog. Cardiovasc. Nurs.,* 2007, 22(2), 72-80.

[107] Palatini, P; Visentin, P; Dorigatti, F; Guarnieri, C; Santonastas, M; Cozzio, S; Pegoraro, F; Bortolazzi, A; Vriz, O; Mos, L. the HARVEST Study Group. Regular physical activity prevents development of left ventricular hypertrophy in hypertension. *Eur. Heart J.,* 2009, 30(2), 225-232.

In: Cardiac Rehabilitaiton
Editor: J. T. Halliday, pp. 99-119

ISBN: 978-1-60741-918-1

Chapter IV

Does Treating Hypertension in the Very Elderly Equally Reduce Mortality in all Subgroups?

Adriano Lubini[1], Jarbas S. Roriz-Filho[2], Idiane Rosset-Cruz[3] and Matheus Roriz-Cruz[4*]

[1]Geriatric Medicine Study Group. Department of Internal Medicine. Brazilian Federal University of Rio Grande do Sul State, Brazil
[2]Division of Geriatrics. Department of Internal Medicine. School of Medicine of Ribeirão Preto at University of São Paulo, Brazil
[3]Division of Gerontological Nursing. Faculty of Nursing. Brazilian Federal University of Rio Grande do Sul State, Brazil
[4]Geriatric Medicine Study Group. Department of Internal Medicine. Brazilian Federal University of Rio Grande do Sul State, Brazil

Abstract

There is already a large body of evidence suggesting that hypertension among the youngest-old (65–80 years-old) should be treated no differently from that of younger adults. This includes the

[*] Corresponding Author: Matheus Roriz-Cruz

current definition of hypertension (≥ 140 mmHg for systolic or ≥ 90 mmHg for diastolic Blood Pressure [BP]) also for this age group. Even though orientations from the 'VII Joint on Hypertension' have recommended the extrapolation of this evidence also for the oldest-old group (≥ 80 y.o), until recently there was no definite evidence that treating hypertension in this age group would reduce overall mortality. In fact, a meta-analysis of several mega clinical trials, which have included small subgroups of very elderly people, has found a reverse relationship between treating hypertension and overall mortality. Very recently, the HyVET study has found that treating otherwise healthy very elderly hypertensive (systolic BP 160–210 mmHg as inclusion criteria) people at a goal of 150 x 80 mmHg of systolic and diastolic BP, respectively, reduces overall mortality over an average 1.8 year period. However, several considerations should arise when interpreting data from this study. First, this study included vastly healthy elderly people, having excluded subjects with heart failure (HF), dementia, and frail, institutionalized, elderly people. HF and dementia are possibly the two main confounders of the relationship between BP and mortality among the very elderly. BP tends to decrease in dilated hypertensive myocardiopathy, as it does in malnutrition states associated with advanced dementia. In fact, a study has found that, in the general very elderly population, hypertension was only associated with increased overall mortality after excluding people who have deceased within a 3-year period from baseline, a disproportional part of them apparently from HF and dementia. Aging is a heterogeneous process, and considering only chronological age may not be adequate in analyzing the relationship between BP and mortality in the very elderly. For instance, the relationship between BP and risk of ischemic stroke is the inverse among people with bilateral carotid stenosis ≥ 70%, regardless of age. As a general rule, it may be reasonable deciding to treat otherwise healthy very elderly hypertensive people (without HF, significant carotid stenosis, or moderate-to-advanced dementia) with at least 2 consecutive systolic BP measures ≥ 160 mmHg. In this specific age group, the therapeutic goal should be 150 x 80 mmHg, as evidenced by the HyVET study. Lower BP levels might be associated with an increased risk of hypoperfusional stroke even among otherwise healthy very elderly people, since cerebral blood flow autoregulation is lost in the presence of significant cerebrovascular disease — a finding not uncommon in this age group.

1. Introduction

World population has continued its transition path from a state of high birth and death rates to one characterized by low birth and death rates, for the first time in the history of the world [1, 2]. As a consequence of this transition, a growth in the number and proportion of older persons has been occurring. According to the United Nations, in the beginning of the 21st century, 10% of the population was 60 years old or above; by 2050, the proportion is expected to be 20% [1].

Moreover, the older population itself is aging. In fact, the proportion of very elderly people (80 years or older) is increasing faster than the other segments of the older population [1]. On a worldwide perspective, they currently represent 11% of the age group older than 60 years and are expected to be up to 19% by 2050. There is an obvious predominance of women among the older population, representing 55% of those above 60 years and 65% of the group older than 80 years [1].

Even though it has occurred first in rich countries and urban populations, population ageing is now a worldwide phenomenon. Indeed, developing regions like Latin America and Southest Asia have currently the most accelerated speed of aging in the world [1].

Hypertension is a very common disease in patients over 65 years-old, and its prevalence increases with age, reaching a proportion higher than 70% among those over 85 years. However, elderly adults, especially those aged 80 and older, have been underrepresented in therapeutic trials (3). Age above 65 years is the strongest risk factor for lacking awareness of having hypertension. In fact, in the United States this is the age group with the higher proportion of uncontrolled hypertension [3].

According to the last (VII) JOINT on Hypertension (2003), definition of hypertension among older subjects is no different from that in younger adults, that is, systolic levels $\geq$ 140 mmHg or diastolic levels $\geq$ 90 mmHg. This classification is based on the mean of 2 or more properly measured seated Blood Pressure (BP) readings on each of 2 or more office visits [4].

2. The Evidence

Among patients younger than 65 years, there is a large body of data evidencing a positive quasi-linear relationship between treating hypertension and subsequent reduction of mortality [5]. Older patients appear to benefit from treatment of hypertension in terms of reduced incidence of stroke, heart failure, and other vascular events as do younger patients. However, this benefit is clearer among the youngest-old, that is, patients between the ages of 65 and 80 years and even so among those with few comorbidities [6].

Among people ≥ 80 years, so-called very elderly, or oldest-old, however, there is much controversy if treating hypertension really reduces overall mortality. Clinical trials which have included this very elderly population have reported conflicting findings. Some studies have found worse survival in patients with systolic Blood Pressure (BP) levels below 140 mmHg [7,8].

The INDANA meta-analysis, conducted in the 1990s, focused on the analysis of subgroups of mega trials that have included very elderly patients with hypertension, It totaled 1670 patients who were randomized either for high doses of a diuretic (other than indapamide) or beta-blockers [9]. The meta-analysis concluded that treatment decreased the incidence of stroke by 34%. Also, rates of major cardiovascular events and heart failure were significantly decreased by 22% and 39%, respectively. However, apparently paradoxically, there was no treatment benefit for cardiovascular death, and there was even an increase in the rate of total mortality by 14% in the treatment group [9].

In 2007, another meta-analysis was published with more than 4000 very elderly patients, including patients with comorbidities such as diabetes mellitus, coronary artery disease, congestive heart failure, cerebrovascular disease, and chronic renal failure [8]. More than 80% of those patients were receiving anti-hypertensives. This study has examined whether or not there was an association between different BP levels and survival. The study did not evidence a linear relationship between BP levels and mortality. However, as in the INDANA meta-analysis, patients whose initial BP was considered to be adequately controlled, that is, levels less than 140/90 mmHg, had lower survival rates than did those with higher BP levels. It was suggested that the extrapolation of results of hypertension studies involving younger patients to the very old might be erroneous and dangerous [9]. Otherwise, this might suggest reverse causality, that is, a very high risk comorbidity would be responsible for BP reduction during treatment and not vice versa. [10].

Before 2008 there was no definite evidence that the treatment of hypertension in the very elderly group would reduce overall mortality. But in that year, the HyVET study— an international, multi-centre, randomised double-blind placebo-controlled study—was published. This study has analysed the treatment of hypertension in patients older than 80 years old who had had a sustained systolic BP of more than 160 mmHg. Randomized patients have received either the diuretic indapamide or placebo. The angiotensin-converting enzyme inhibitor perindopril or a placebo were added if necessary. The target BP in the HyVET was 150/80 mmHg. The inclusion criteria were systolic BP between 160 and 210 mmHg, and diastolic BP of less than 110 mmHg. This study had 3845 patients who underwent randomization to receive active treatment or placebo. The exclusion criteria of the study were hemorrhagic stroke in the previous 6 months, heart failure, serum creatinine level greater than 150 μmol per liter (1.7 mg/dL), serum potassium level lower than 3.5 or higher than 5.5 mmol/L, gout, diagnosis of clinical dementia, and being institutionalized [11]. In the authors' view, this high number of exclusion criteria is the major practical limitation of the study, since most subjects might have been excluded. This makes extrapolations of results to the general very elderly population difficult. Moreover, a major methodological flaw is the fact that is not clear how many patients were excluded at baseline from the HyVET, since the initial sample was not informed. These issues are further discussed below.

That said, the HyVET study has evidenced beneficial use of the antihypertensive treatment of indapamide, with or without perindopril, compared with the placebo group. The endpoint which was most favourably influenced by treatment was heart failure, as related below:

- Reduction in the rate of heart failure: 64%
- Reduction in the rate of fatal stroke: 39%
- Reduction in the rate of stroke: 30%
- Reduction in the rate of mortality for any cause: 21%
- Reduction in the rate of any cardiovascular event (death from any cardiovascular cause, including stroke, myocardial infarction, and heart failure): 34%.

There was a difference of 15.0/6.1 mmHg in systolic and diastolic BP, respectively, between the active- and placebo-treatment groups at 2 years of follow-up. After 2 years, the target BP of 150X80 mmHg was reached in nearly 50% of the subjects in the intervention group. The number necessary to treat (NNT) to prevent 1 stroke and 1 fatal event for any cause were respectively, 94 and 40 in 2 years [11].

To date, the HyVET study is the only investigation specifically designed to evaluate whether or not it is worth treating hypertension in this age group. Notwithstanding this merit, as mentioned above, it is necessary to consider its limitations, especially the fact that its very elderly sample was especially healthy, since the HyVET excluded not only institutionalized subjects and those with dementia, but also those with heart failure and other comorbidities.

3. Concerns about the Treatment of Hypertension in the Very Elderly

Many causative directions are involved in the relationship between midlife hypertension, atherosclerosis, cerebral small-vessel disease, brain hypoperfusion, neurodegeneration, and dementia, including Alzheimer's disease (Figure 1).

Boxes with solid lines represent risk factors for cognitive dysfunction. Boxes with dashed lines represent possible pathophysiological pathways linking these risk factors cerebral hypoperfusion and dementia, including Alzheimer´s disease (adapted from reference 12).

3.1. Dementia

There are many lines of evidence to suggest that hypertension raises the risk not only of vascular dementia, but also of Alzheimer-type [13]. Involved mechanisms in this later causation process are not completely understood, but seem to involve chronic damage to the endothelium of the cerebral microcirculation. Notwithstanding, hypotension is also associated with dementia, and many physicians are concerned that aggressive treatment of hypertension may cause cerebral hypoperfusion and associated syncope, falls, or cognitive dysfunction. This apparent discrepancy is reflected by some studies which have evidenced a U-shaped curve between BP levels and risk for dementia [14]. This phenomenon possibly occurs due to a chronic condition of cerebral hypoperfusion, suggesting that, in some cases, higher BP levels might be necessary to guarantee adequate cerebral perfusion [14].

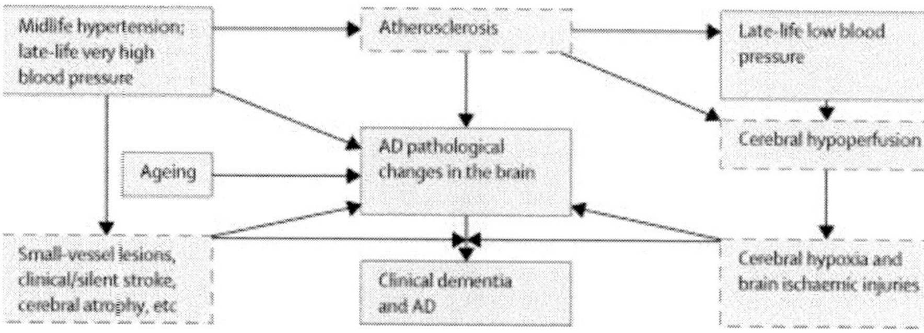

Figure 1. Causative directions involved in the relationship between midlife hypertension, atherosclerosis, late-life low blood pressure, cerebral small-vessel disease, brain hypoperfusion, neurodegeneration, and dementia, including Alzheimer's disease.

Elderly people often have different degrees of carotid obstruction, and some studies have suggested that it is this degree of stenosis, and not necessarily chronological age by itself, which requires higher mean BP levels in order to keep adequate cerebral perfusion pressures [15]. In fact, among people with bilateral carotid stenosis $\geq 70\%$, lower BP levels are associated with increased risk of stroke [15]. However, a study conducted among otherwise healthy elderly hypertensive subjects has found that, after 6 months follow-up, hypertensive subjects that have controlled their BP levels had significant increases in carotid distensibility and cerebral blood flow velocity in the middle cerebral artery, when compared with their uncontrolled BP counterparts [16]. Taken together, these studies suggest that antihypertensive therapy may improve cerebral perfusion and carotid artery distensibility in healthy hypertensive subjects, i.e., before a significant degree of carotid stenosis develops and the brain's blood flow autoregulatory capacity is lost.

Besides, moderate to advanced dementing states are associated with weight loss and, eventually, decreased BP levels. In fact, some studies even suggest that elderly people who will develop dementia may start to lose weight still in the preclinical stages of the dementing process [17].

3.2. Depression

Hypertension is a risk factor for cardiovascular diseases and both symptomatic and asymptomatic stroke and, indirectly, could be a risk for depression. However, many studies, have suggested that depressive disorder among older people is associated with lower systolic BP levels [18,19,20]. In a follow-up study with more than 1,000 patients with mean age of 65 years, lower BP levels were associated with 2 years higher incidence of depressive symptomatology [21]. The possibility of an inverse causation process, i.e., that baseline depressive symptoms may be associated with lower BP levels after 2 years of follow-up did not prove to be true. A hypothesis is that low BP itself causes depression, through increasing somatic symptoms, fatigue and affecting physical and social activities [21]. Other hypotheses are that chronic cerebral hypoperfusion may lead to disorders in the central monoamine activity and to both neurodegeneration (Alzheimer's disease) and micro-infarcts (vascular dementia and depression).

Even though confounding factors do not seem to completely explain the relationship between depression and low BP, the possibility of its occurrence should be investigated when an elderly person presents with both morbidities. In fact, some antihypertensive drugs may lead to higher depressive symptomatology (β-blocker, α-methyldopa, clonidine, calcium channels blockers, reserpine), whereas the use of certain antidepressants is associated with both high diastolic and systolic BPs and hypertension [21].

3.3. Cardiovascular Diseases

As a consequence of some structural and functional alterations which may occur in the cardiovascular system as people age, very elderly subjects have much high prevalences of cardiovascular disorders which may affect BP levels. [7] Studies with this age group have shown lower BP levels in patients with previous history of myocardial infarction, heart failure or stroke. Hypotension has been interpreted as a marker of both geriatric frailty and some advanced disease processes like heart failure, dementia, Patients with heart failure secondary to dilated myocardiopathy usually have lower BP levels. Those patients are at the highest risk for mortality [22].

3.4. Carotid Stenosis

The relationship between systolic BP and risk of stroke is inverse among subjects with bilateral carotid stenosis ($\geq$ 70%), i.e., the lower the BP, the higher the incidence of stroke [15]. Individuals with unilateral carotid stenosis have the lowest risk of stroke at systolic BP levels of 150 mmHg, the risk increasing in a U-like fashion at lower or higher BP levels.

The prevalence of uni- or bilateral carotid stenosis among the elderly population is about 5%. In the presence of brain ischemia, cerebral autoregulatory capacity is lost (Figure 2). At normal situations, Normaly, there is an autoregulatory plateau with mean arterial BP values between 50 e 150 mmHg, when cerebral blood flow is optimal. Under cerebral ischemic conditions, however, cerebral blood flow depends directly on the perfusion pressure. Cerebral blood flow usually has its autoregulatory capacity restored after carotid endarterectomy. Taken together, these data suggest that aggressive treatment of hypertension in subjects with carotid stenosis may be harmful. In this case, revascularization should be done prior to treatment of hypertension [15].

3.5. Blood Pressure Target

It is unclear whether treating very elderly subjects with BP levels lower than 150/80 mmHg would have benefits, even among the healthiest ones. Indeed, lower BP targets among healthy very-elderly individuals were not analyzed until presently. It would not be adequate to extrapolate the results of the HyVET to frail patients [11].

Please note that autoregulation is lost in conditions of cerebral ischemia (including chronic ischemic states). Note that the plateau is deviated to the left among hypertensive subjects, but the brain autoregulatory capacity is not lost. For this reason, treatment of hypertension among very-elderly hypertensive subjects should start at low doses and doses should be escalated only slowly, as the plateau moves to the left with time with readaptation to the new cerebral perfusion pressures. Adapted from reference 23.

3.6. Isolated Systolic Blood Pressure

Among the oldest-old there is a very high prevalence of isolated systolic BP [24]. Before 50 years of age it is more frequent elevated diastolic BP. After this age, systolic pressure continues to rise but diastolic BP tends to fall. Consequently, isolated systolic hypertension predominates among older persons [24]. This occurs because aging and atherosclerosis reduce the elasticity and compliance of large arteries [25]. However, studies that documented physicians' behavior confirmed that doctors are unlikely to diagnose persistently elevated systolic pressure with a diastolic pressure of less than 90 mm Hg as hypertension, or avoid treating this condition aggressively [4].

The VII Joint National Committee guidelines, recommends thiazide-type diuretics as the initial drug therapy for most patients with isolated systolic hypertension. The use of a dihydropyridine calcium channel blocker was also recommended as beneficial in the isolated systolic hypertension of the elderly [4,26,27].

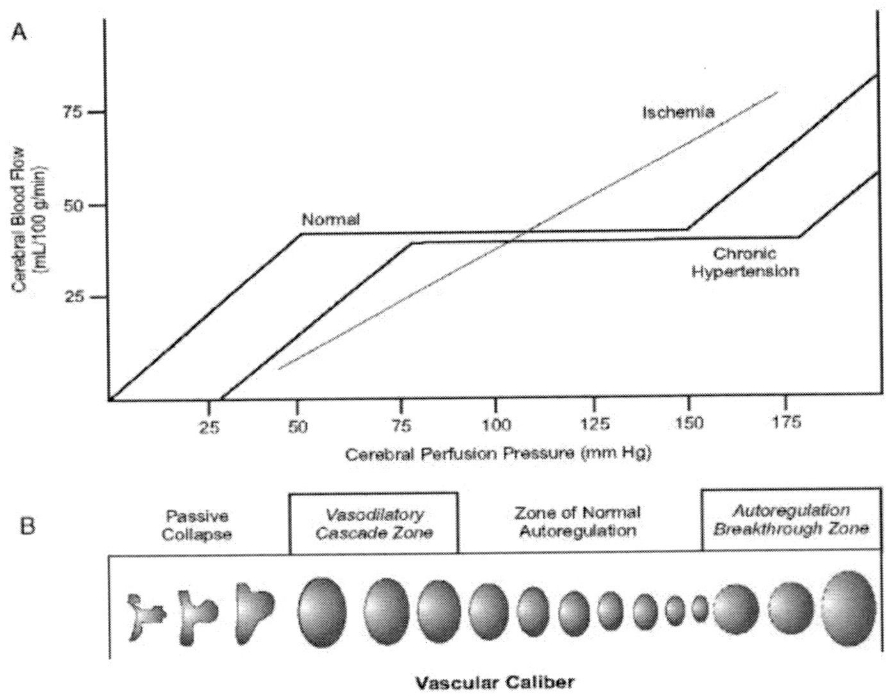

Figure 2. A. Relationship between Cerebral Perfusion Pressure and Cerebral Blood Flow in situations of normality, chronic hypertension, and chronic brain ischemia states; B. Arterial caliber according to the different stages of cerebral autoregulation.

3.7. Pulse Pressure

Pulse pressure is the difference between systolic and diastolic BP. A very recent study has shown that higher levels of pulse pressure were independently associated with a higher incidence of atrial fibrillation, with a cumulative 20-year incidence rate of 5.6% for pulse pressure of 40 mm Hg or less and 23.3% for pulse pressure greater than 61 mm Hg [28,29]. An elevated pulse pressure is also associated with higher incidence of dilatation of left atrium, impaired ventricular relaxation, heart failure, and myocardial infarction in normotensive and hypertensive persons [30]. Age, diabetes mellitus, and hypertension are also associated with conduit artery stiffness, and hence are also risk factors for the elevation of pulse pressure [31].

An excessive reduction of diastolic pressure could be dangerous in those with coronary artery disease because myocardial perfusion occurs during the diastole [32]. The SHEP study has evidenced an increased risk of cardiovascular disease at levels of diastolic BP < 70 mm Hg, but this effect was more important diastolic BP levels dropped below 60 mm Hg [33,34].

3.8. Postural Hypotension

A very important concern in the initiation of antihypertensive treatment among the oldest-old is the higher risk of postural hypotension. For this reason, it is imperative measuring BP in the recumbent, sitting, and standing positions. Long-standing postural BP fluctuation may impair cerebral perfusion and promotes changes such as lacunes and leukoaraiosis [35]. If lacunae happens also in the medulla oblongata, this might creates a vicious circle as they might disrupt brainstem's vasomotor center, essential for prompt postural BP control [35,36] Some studies have found poorer scores on neurobehavioral tests and cognitive decline among elderly patients with postural hypotension [36]. Postural hypotension is more frequent in older patients with systolic hypertension, diabetes, neurological diseases, and those taking cardiovascular medications such as diuretics, venodilators (nitrates, α-blockers, and drugs for the treatment of erectile dysfunction, such as sildenafil), besides some psychotropic drugs with anticholinergic effects. In these subjects, it is important to avoid iatrogenic volume depletion caused by the use of high dose diuretics. If the antihypertensive treatment is absolutely necessary, main doses of should be given at bedtime.

Therefore, it is important for the physician to remember that postural hypotension should always be investigated among very elderly patients. Attention should be duplicated if these elderly subjects have also other associated risk factors for postural hypotension, such as is the case in alcoholics, diabetics, Parkinsonians, demented subjects, and those with heart failure. Postural hypotension should also always be looked for in patients presenting with dizziness, syncope, or postural palpitations/tachycardia. Again, it is important here to avoid volume depletion and excessively rapid dose titration of antihypertensive drugs [4].

4. Treatment and Rehabilitation

Like any hypertensive patient, the initial evaluation of the oldest-old should be focused on defining the severity of hypertension, the investigation of possible secondary causes, and the identification of other risk factors for cardiovascular diseases. The VII Joint recommends a complete anamnesis and physical examination, serum chemistry screen, simple urine exam, and an electrocardiogram for the initial evaluation. [4]

Both pharmacological and non-pharmacological management of hypertension and hypertensive myocardiopathy in the very elderly are intended not only to reduce lesions at target-organs and mortality, but also to contribute in ***cardiac rehabilitation*** by reducing concentric myocardial hypertrophy and its consequences, like diastolic dysfunction and fatal and non-fatal arrhythmias.

4.1. Pharmacological Management

The treatment with thiazide type-diuretic or indapamide, as shown in the HyVET study, is very beneficial and should be the first choice in treating hypertension also in the very. In patients with hypertension and chronic kidney disease, it is recommend the use of an ACE inhibitor or an angiotensin-receptor blocker. A study published in 2005 has shown that the use of a β – blocker as a monotherapy is suboptimal as it was associated with a substantially higher risk of stroke than treatment with other antihypertensive agents used in mnonotherapy. Therefore, the use of other class agents is recommended. Notwithstanding, this is not the case when hypertension is associated with congestive heart failure, some types of arrhythmias, coronary arterial disease, and increased sympathetic activity. In all these situations a β-blocker is most possibly benefical [37, 38]. A calcium channel blocker can also be recommended in these patients as well, especially in patients with angina who have a formal contraindication for the use of β-blocker.

In the very elderly and, specially, the more frail patients, initial doses and subsequent dose titration should be more gradual because of a greater chance of undesirable side effects [10]. It is very important to remember that elderly subjects may be more prone to electrolytic disturbances caused by antihypertensives such as diuretics and ACE inhibitors, which can cause hypokalemia and hyperkalemia, respectively. Very elderly subjects are also more prone to arrhythmias and even sudden death in the presence of electrolytic abnormalities, such as hyperkalemia. The association between these classes of anti-hypertensives, as tested in the HyVET study, could have a neutral effect in potassium levels [11].

4.2. Non-Pharmacological Management

Besides the pharmacological management of high BP, lifestyle measures have no reasons not to be also instituted in elderly patients. They have proved not only to low BP levels, but also have been shown to control other atherosclerotic risk factors. Besides, these measures have also the objective of reducing the posology of antihypertensive drugs.

- Increase in fruit and vegetable intake and decrease in saturated and total fat intake.

The study 'Dietary Approaches to Stop Hypertension (DASH) ' trial demonstrated that a diet rich in fruits, vegetables, and fibers, and poor intake of red meats, sweets, total and saturated fat, and cholesterol lowers BP significantly when compared with a typical western diet. According to that study, there is a reduction in systolic BP levels by 8 to 14 mmHg, an effect similar to single drug therapy. However, these evidences were shown in younger populations, with mean age of 54.7 years, and there has not been large-scale trials on the impact of diet modification among elderly adults [39].

A Mediterranean diet with a moderate amount of fat and a high proportion of monounsaturated fat (rich in vegetables and low in red meat, with poultry and fish, olive oil and nuts) provides cardiovascular benefits and its value is generally accepted for all age groups . A study has shown a loss of 4.4 kg and favorable changes in fasting plasma glucose, lipoproteins metabolism, and insulin levels with a Mediterranean diet modification program [40]. Hypertensive patients should be advised to eat more fruits and vegetables (4–5 servings per day), to prefer fish instead of read meat, to ingest complex carbohydrates with low glycemic index (which are less absorved by the intestin, being associated with inferior secretion of insuline), and to reduce intake of saturated fat and cholesterol.

- *Smoking cessation.* Smoking acts as a risk factor for hypertension through its atherosclerotic effect. Moreover, smoking is a powerful independent cardiovascular risk factor, and smoking cessation is probably the single most effective lifestyle measure for the prevention of myocardial infarction [10]. Hypertensive smokers should be counseled regarding smoking cessation. Pharmacological treatment sometimes can be considered [41].
- *Reduction of salt intake.* Reducing sodium intake by 80–100mmol (4.7–5.8 g of sodium chloride) per day from an initial intake of around 180mmol (10.5 g of sodium chloride) per day reduce BP by an average of 4–6mmHg [4]. That effect is even more important when associated with other dietary measures. An excessive intake of salt may be the cause of a resistant hypertensive status. The maximum recommended daily intake sodium is less than 5 g/day of sodium chloride (85mmol/day). Patients must avoid adding salt in food and they should also be disencouraged in routinely eating processed food. The effect of sodium restriction on BP is even greater among elderly patients due to the less responsiveness of the renin-angiotensin-aldosterone system [42].
- *Reduction of excessive alcohol intake.* Consume of low doses of alcoholic drinks (up to two daily doses for men and one dose for women) results in reduced BP (mean reduction of 2-4 mmHg in systolic BP) and total mortality compared to non-drinkers. However, heavy drinkers have more elevated BP levels and higher incidence of stroke and total mortality. Most studies have found that the nadir of the mortality curve is situated between the daily doses of ethanol of

20-30g for men and 10–20g for women [43]. However, patients who do not drink should not be incentived to drink, since the potential adverse effects of individual cases of alcoholism may outstand the small beneficial outcome in any group.

- *Physical exercise.* Regular exercise provides many benefits for older adults, including improvements in BP, diabetes, lipid profile, osteoarthritis, osteoporosis, neurocognitive function, improved quality of sleep and lower risk of depression, fatigue and chronic pain [44] Mean reduction in resting BP with a program of physical exercise conduced among younger hypertensive patients was 6.9/ for systolic BP and 4.9mmHg for diastolic BP [4] Engaged subjects have also reduced body weight, body fat and waist circumference, and increased insulin sensitivity and HDL-cholesterol levels. However, up to 75% of the older adult population does not currently exercise at recommended levels [44]. Few contraindications to exercise exist (recent ECG change or myocardial infarction, unstable angina, third-degree heart block, acute congestive heart failure, uncontrolled hypertension or metabolic disease)[44]. Almost all older persons can benefit from additional physical activity. Sedentary patients should be advised to take up exercise of moderate intensity for at least 30 minutes, most days of the week [4, 10].
- *Weight reduction and weight stabilization.* Studies have shown that body weight is directly associated with hypertension and weight reduction lowers BP in obese patients. Obviously, weight reduction has beneficial effects on associated risk factors (insulin resistance, diabetes, hyperlipidemia, left ventricular hypertrophy, and obstructive sleep apnea). In a study, the reduction of BP with an average weight loss of 5.1 kg was 4.4 mmHg for systolic pressure and 3.6mmHg for diastolic BP [4, 45].

5. Conclusions

In conclusion, the evidence up till now published in the medical literature about the treatment of hypertension in the very elderly can be summarized as follows:

- It is reasonable to treat otherwise healthy very elderly hypertensive patients (with at least 2 consecutive systolic BP measures greater than 160 mmHg). The therapeutic goal should be 150 X 80 mmHg, as evidenced in the HyVET study. The benefit from lower targets still needs to be established. Since there is no definitive evidence, demented or institutionalized patients, those with heart failure, significant carotid stenosis or history of recent stroke should be evaluated case-to-case on an individual basis. It might be reasonable to consider treatment in these cases if systolic BP is above 175–180 mmHg. Especially in these cases, the old rule 'start low and go slowly' should not be forgotten. In these situations, a reasonable target systolic BP would be around 160–165 mmHg.
- The drug of first choice in this age group should be a thiazide-type diuretic, which, if necessary, may be associated with an angiotensin-converting-enzyme (ACE) inhibitor. Another option is the use of angiotensin II receptor antagonists (***ARA II), particularly in patients which are intolerant to the use of ACE inhibitors.*** It is important that the evaluation of postural hypotension be done before starting anti-hypertensive drugs in this age group. If the antihypertensive treatment is absolutely necessary, main doses should be given at bedtime.
- Lower BP levels might be associated with an increased risk of hypoperfusional stroke, since cerebral blood flow auto-regulation is lost in the presence of significant cerebrovascular disease (finding not uncommon in very elderly patients), including significant carotid stenosis.
- A successful and well-tolerated therapy must not be interrupted when a patient reaches 80 years of age. It is reasonable to keep former medications and to periodically evaluate their need. Sometimes it might even be necessary to increase antihypertensive doses, or to add new drugs in order to control BP. The presence of subclinical organ damage and comorbities (such as clinical cardiovascular disease, renal disease, or diabetes) is also important in choosing the more appropriate drug for each case [10].
- Aging is a very complex phenomenon and a heterogeneous process. Individuals become more dissimilar as they age. Therefore, since there is no clinical marker of biological ageing, considering only chronological age might not be adequate in analyzing the relationship between BP and mortality in this age group. Medical literature on the

subject is poor. Therefore, since hypertension treatment decisions in these patients are frequently unclear, the decision whether to lower BP is frequently challenging. Doctors and patients should balance benefits against risks, sharing and agreeing in the final treatment decision [34].

- The prevention, early diagnosis, treatment and rehabilitation of other associated pathologies, like diabetes, heart failure, and dyslipidemia should always be intended. Modifying lifestyle, abandoning tobacco, and avoiding excessive alcohol consumption are, along with other non-pharmacological measures, all important measures in controlling BP as well.

Rehabilitation from hypertension-related concentric hypertrophic myocardiopathy and frequently associated diastolic heart failure requires an approach which involves not only a long-term control of hypertension in the very elderly, but also an aerobic rehabilitation program.

References

[1] United Nations. Report of the Second World Assembly on Aging. Madrid, Spain: United Nations, April, 8-12, 2002.

[2] Escovitz, GH. The Health Transition in Developing Countries: A Role for Internists from the Developed World. *Annals of Internal Medicine,* 1992, 116, 499-504.

[3] Haijar, I. Kotchen, Trends in prevalence, awareness, treatment and control of hypertension in the United States. *JAMA,* 2003, 290, 199-203.

[4] Chobanian, AV; Barkis, GL; Black, HR; et al. The seventh report of the National Committee on Prevention, Detection, Evaluation and Treatment of High Blood Pressure. The JNC 7 Report. *JAMA.*, 2003, 289, 2560-2572.

[5] Messerli, F; Williams, B; Ritz, E. Essencial hypertension. *The Lancet*, 2007, 370, 591-603.

[6] Rastas, Sari Association Between Blood Pressure and Survival over 9 Year in a General Population Aged 85 and Older. *J Am Geriatr Soc* 54:912-918, 2006.

[7] Goodwin, J. Embracing complexity: A consideration of hypertension in the very old. *J Gerontol A Biol Sci Med Sci,* 2003, 58A, M653-M658.

[8] Oates, DJ. et al. Blood pressure and survival in the oldest old. *J Am Geriatrics Society*, 2007, 55, 383-388

[9] Gueyffier, et al.Antihypertensive drugs in very old people: a subgroup meta-analysis of randomised controlled trials. *THE LANCET* • Vol 353 • March, 6, 1999.

[10] Mancia, G; De Backer, G; et al. Guidelines for the Management of Arterial Hypertension.The Task Force for the Management of Arterial Hypertension of the European Society of Hypertension (ESH) and of the European Society of Cardiology (ESC). *Journal of Hypertension,* 2007, 25, 1105-1187.

[11] Beckett, NS; Peters, R; Fletcher, AE; Staessen, JA; Liu, L; Dumitrascu, D; Stoyanovsky, V; Antikainen, RL; Nikitin, Y; Anderson, C; Belhani, A; Forette, F; Chakravarthi, R; Thijs, L; Banya, W; Bulpitt, CJ. Treatment of Hypertension in Patients 80 years of age or older. *The New England Journal of Medicine.*, 2008, Vol 358 No 18, 1887-1898.

[12] Qiu, C; Winblad Qiu, C; Winblad, B; FratiglionL.The age-dependent relation of blood pressure to cognitive function and dementia. *Lancet Neurol,* 2005, 4, 487-99.

[13] Forette, F; Seux, M. L; Staessen, J; Thijs, K; Babarskiene, M. R; Babeanu, S; Bossini, A; Fagard, R; Gil-Extremera, B; Laks, T; Kobalava, Z; Sarti, C; Tuomilehto, J; Vanhanen, H; Webster, J; Yodfat, Y; Birkenhager, W. The prevention of dementia with antihypertensive treatment. New evidence from the systolic hypertension in Europe (Syst-Eur) study. *Archives of Internal Medicine.*, 2002, 162, 2046-2052.

[14] Guo, Z; Viitanen, M; Fratiglioni, L; Winblad, B. Low blood pressure and dementia in elderly people: the Kungsholmen project. *BMJ,* 1996, 312, 805-08

[15] Rothwell, PM; Howard, SC; Spence, JD. Relationship Between Blood Pressure and Stroke Risk in Patients With Symptomatic Carotid Occlusive Disease. *Stroke*, 2003, 34, 2583-2592.

[16] Lipsitz, LA; Gagnon, M; Vyas, M; Iloputaife, I; Kiely, DK; Sorond, F; Serrador, J; Cheng, DM; Babikian, V; Cupples, LA. Antihypertensive Therapy Increases Cerebral Blood Flow and Carotid Distensibility in Hypertensive Elderly Subject. *Hypertension*, 2004, 44, 625-630.

[17] Johnson, DK; Wilkins, CH; Morris, JC. Accelerated Weight Loss May Precede Diagnosis in Alzheimer Disease. *Archives of Neurology,* 2006, 63, 1312-1317.

[18] Licht, CMM; Geus, EJC; Seldenrijk, A; van Hout, HPJ; Zitman, FG; van Dyck, R; Penninx, BWJH. Depression Is Associated With Decreased Blood Pressure, but Antidepressant Use Increases the Risk for Hypertension. *Hypertension*, 2009, 53, 631-638

[19] Wessely, S; Nickson, J; Cox, B. Symptoms of low blood pressure: a population study. *British Medical Journal,* 1990, 301, 18-25

[20] Pilgrim, JA; Stansfeld, S; Marmot, M. Low blood pressure low mood. *British Medical Journal,* 1992, 304, 75-78

[21] Paterniti, S; Verdier-Taillefer, MH; Geneste, C; Bisserbe, JC; Alperovitch, A. Low blood pressure and risk of depression in the elderly. A prospective community-based study. *British Journal of Psychiatry*. 2000, 176, 464-467.

[22] Gheorghiade, M; Abraham, WT; Albert, NM, et al. Systolic Blood Pressure at Admission, Clinical Characteristics, and Outcomes in patients Hospitalized With Acute Heart Failure. *JAMA*, 2006, Vol 296, No. 18, 2216 - 2227

[23] Varon, J. Diagnosis and management of labile blood pressure during acute cerebrovascular accidents and other hypertensive crises. *American Journal of Emergency Medicine,* 2007, 25, 949-959.

[24] Lewington, S; Clarke, R; Qizilbash, N; Peto, R; Collins, R. Age-specific relevance of usual blood pressure to vascular mortality: a meta-analysis of individual data for one million adults in 61 prospective studies. *Lancet*, 2002, 360, 1903-13.

[25] Zieman, SJ; Melenovsky, V; Kass, DA. Mechanisms, pathophysiology, and therapy of arterial stiffness. *Arterioscler Thromb Vasc Biol*, 2005, 25, 932-43.

[26] Liu, L; Wang, JL; Gong, L; Liu, G; Staessen, JA. for the Syst-China Collaborative Group .Comparison of active treatment and placebo in older Chinese patients with isolated systolic hypertension. *Journal of Hypertension*, 1998, 16, 1823-1829.

[27] Papademetriou, V; Farsang, C; et al. Study on Cognition and Prognosis in the Elderly study group. Stroke prevention with the angiotensin II type 1-receptor blocker candesartan in elderly patients with isolated systolic hypertension: the Study on Cognition and Prognosis in the Elderly (SCOPE). *J Am Coll Cardiol*, 2004, 44, 1175-1180.

[28] Blacher, J; Staessen, JA; Girerd, X; et al. Pulse pressure not mean pressure determines cardiovascular risk in older hypertensive patients. *Arch InternMed*. 2000, 160, 1085-1089.

[29] Mitchel, et al. Pulse Pressure and Risk of New-Onset Atrial Fibrillation. *JAMA,* 2007, 297(7), 709-715

[30] Haider, AW et al. Systolic Blood Pressure, Diastolic Blood Pressure, and Pulse Pressure as Predictors of Risk for Congestive Heart Failure in the Framingham Heart Study. *Ann Intern Med*, 2003, 7, 138(1), 10-6.

[31] Franklin, SS; Khan, SA; Wong, ND; Larson, MG; Levy, D. Is pulse pressure useful in predicting risk for coronary heart Disease? The Framingham heart study. *Circulation.*, 1999, 100, 354-60.

[32] Messerli, FH; Mancia, G; Conti, CR; et al. Dogma disputed: can aggressively lowering blood pressure in hypertensive patients with coronary artery disease be dangerous? *Ann Intern Med*, 2006, 144, 884-93

[33] Somes, GW; Pahor, M; Shorr, RI; Cushman, WC. The role of diastolic blood pressure when treating isolated systolic hypertension. *Arch Intern Med*. 1999, 159, 2004-2009.

[34] Chaudhry, Sarwat.; Krumholz, Harlan; Foody, JoAnne Systolic Hypertension in Older Persons. *JAMA,* 2004;292(9):1074-1080 JAMA

[35] Helenius, J; Soinne, L; Salonen, O; Kaste, M; Tatlisumak, T. Leukoaraiosis, Ischemic Stroke, and Normal White Matter on Diffusion-Weighted MRI.

[36] Matsubayashi, K; Okumiya, K; Wada, T; Osaki, Y; Fujisawa, M; Doi, Y; Ozawa, T. Postural disregulation in systolic blood pressure is associated with worsened score in neurobehavioral functional tests and leukoaraiosis in the older living in older elderly living in a community. *Stroke,* 1997, 28, 2169 - 2173

[37] Lindholm, LH; Carlberg, B; Samuelson, O. Should β blockers remain first choice in the treatment of primary hypertension? *Lancet*, 2005, 366, 1545-53

[38] Psaty, BM; Lumley, T; Furberg, CD; et al. Health outcomes associated with various antihypertensive therapies used as first-line agents: a network analysis. *JAMA*, 2003, 289, 2534-44.

[39] Appel, LJ; Moore, TJ; Obarzanek, E; et al. A clinical trial of the effects of dietary patterns on blood pressure: DASH Collaborative Research Group. *New England Journal of Medicine*. 1997, 336, 1117-1124.

[40] Shai, I, Schwarzfuchs, D; Henkin Y; et al. Weight Loss with a Low-Carbohydrate, Mediterranean, or Low-Fat Diet. *The New England Journal of Medicine*, 2008, 359, 229-241

[41] Primatesta, P; Falaschetti, E; Gupta, S; Marmot, MG; Poulter, NR. Association between smoking and blood pressure: evidence from the health survey for England. *Hypertension,* 2001, 37, 187-193.

[42] Appel, LJ; Brands, MW; Daniels, SR; Karanja, N; Elmer, PJ; Sacks, FM. American Heart Association. Dietary approaches to prevent and treat hypertension: a scientific statement from the American Heart Association. *Hypertension,* 2006, 47, 296-308.

[43] Rimm, EB; Williams, P; Fosher, K; Criqui, M; Stampfer, MJ. Moderate alcohol intake and lower risk of coronary heart disease: meta-analysis of effects on lipids and haemostatic factors. *British Medical Journal,* 1999, 319, 1523-1528.

[44] Nied, R; Franklin, B. American Family Physician Promoting and Prescribing Exercise for the Elderly. *American Family Physician*, 2002, 65, 421-426

[45] Neter, JE; Stam, BE, Kok, FJ; Grobbee, DE; Geleijnse, JM. Influence of weight reduction on blood pressure: a meta-analysis of randomized controlled trials. *Hypertension,* 2003, 42, 878-884.

In: Cardiac Rehabilitaiton
Editor: J. T. Halliday, pp. 121-141

ISBN: 978-1-60741-918-1

Chapter V

Cardiac Rehabilitation

Kaatje Goetschalckx[(1)] ***and Robert Fagard***[(1,2)*]
[(1)]Cardiovascular Rehabilitation Unit, Department of Cardiology, University Hospital K.U. Leuven and
[(2)]Hypertension and Cardiovascular Rehabilitation Unit, Faculty of Medicine, K.U.Leuven University, Leuven, Belgium

Definition of Cardiac Rehabilitation

In 1993, the World Health Organization (WHO) defined cardiac rehabilitation as the 'sum of activity and interventions required to ensure the best possible physical, mental, and social conditions so that patients with chronic or postacute cardiovascular disease may, by their own efforts, preserve or resume their proper place in society and lead an active life' .

In addition to this definition of rehabilitation as 'restorement', different aspects of the rehabilitation program have shown to have a positive impact on prognosis. Simultaneously terminology has in many settings evolved to 'cardiac rehabilitation and prevention'.

* Corresponding author: University of Leuven, Hypertension Unit, U.Z. Gasthuisberg, Herestraat 49 B-3000 Leuven, Belgium, Tel: 32/16/34.87.07, Fax: 32/16/34.37.66, E-mail: <robert.fagard@ uz.kuleuven.ac.be>

Cardiac Rehabilitation as a Comprehensive Intervention

From an isolated exercise training program, cardiac rehabilitation has evolved to a multidisciplinary comprehensive intervention. [1,2,3] The disciplines involved are represented by a cardiologist specialized in cardiac rehabilitation, a physical therapist, a dietician, a psychologist/occupational therapist and a social worker or social nurse.

In this multidisciplinary approach, an appropriate cardiovascular risk evaluation is made and optimal medical or interventional treatment offered to the patient. This task is traditionally performed by the treating cardiologist, but task overlap exists with the cardiac rehabilitation specialist, watching over all aspects of cardiovascular prevention and prognosis of the patient.

Exercise training is offered as an adjuvant and important component of treatment of cardiovascular diseases.

Education and counselling is performed to achieve risk reduction and life style changes. It involves the application of behavioural treatment strategies and the involvement of family members where appropriate. It includes also vocational counselling.

Adequate follow-up is required to assure long-term compliance.

Clinical Indications for Cardiac Rehabilitation

In secondary prevention, the evidence for a benefit of a cardiac rehabilitation program on mortality, morbidity and quality of life is largest for patients with ischemic heart disease. On the other hand, cardiac rehabilitation has not shown to be harmful in any particular patient population or cardiac disease, apart from the contra-indications listed below. Therefore, as a non-extensive list of clinical indications for cardiac rehabilitation we mention following cardiovascular diseases: after myocardial infarction, CABG, PCI, valve surgery, ICD-implantation, heart transplantation or surgical intervention for a congenital or acquired malformation of the heart, or in patients with stable angina, chronic heart failure or a cardiomyopathy with dysfunction of the left ventricle.

Contra-Indications

The contra-indications for regular physical exercise training are the same as for exercise testing: acute myocardial infarction <2days, unstable angina with recent rest pain, untreated life-threatening cardiac arrhythmias, uncompensated congestive heart failure, uncontrolled hypertension, advanced atrioventricular block, acute myocarditis and pericarditis, symptomatic aortic stenosis, severe hypertrophic obstructive cardiomyopathy, acute pulmonary embolism/pulmonary infarction, acute aortic dissection, acute systemic illness.

Benefit versus Safety Aspects of Regular Physical Exercise Therapy in Secondary Prevention

In a randomized clinical trial of 101 male patients with stable coronary artery disease (angina CCS class I-III due to a significant coronary artery stenosis, with exclusion of acute coronary syndromes, myocardial infarction etc.), exercise training was compared to PCI-treatment. After 12 months, exercise was associated with an increased maximal oxygen uptake of 16% (from 22.7±0.7 to 26.2±0.8 mL $V0_2$/kg/min; $p<0.001$ versus baseline, $p<0.001$ versus PCI group). In addition, it resulted in superior event-free survival (80% versus 70%, $p=0.023$) at lower costs, compared with PCI-treatment. [4] In a meta-analysis of 48 randomized controlled trials of 8940 patients in total (after myocardial infarction, PCI, CABG, angina, known CAD), a structured exercise program was calculated to result in a 20% reduction of total mortality and a 26% reduction in cardiac mortality. [5]

On the other hand, based on a large clinical database of 1960 to 1977, starting a training program in selected patients with known CAD is expected to result in approximately 1 cardiac arrest per 32 593 patient training hours (PTH), 1 cardiac death per 116 402 PTH and 1 myocardial infarction per 232 805 PTH, decreasing to 1 cardiac arrest per 111 996 PTH, 1 cardiac death per 783 972 PHT and 1 myocardial infarction per 293 990 PHT in a later database from 1980 to 1984. [6,7]

In patients with stable chronic heart failure due to ischaemic heart disease (mean left ventricular ejection fraction 19%), peak oxygen uptake increases from 14.3 ml/kg/min to 16.7 ml/kg/min by 8 weeks of home-based bicycle exercise training [8] or ca. 17% by regular exercise training according to a review of 81 studies in 2387 patients.[9] Additionally, exercise training resulted in improved quality of life, with a significant improvement in patient-rated symptom scores, such as tiredness ($p < 0.01$) or breathlessness ($p < 0.05$). [8,10,11].

The results of the EXTRA-MATCH meta-analysis of the ESC with a total of 801 CHF patients documented a significant reduction of total mortality by 35% (odds ratio 0.65, CI 0.46-0.92, P=0.015), and of hospitalization by 28% (odds ratio 0.72, CI 0.56-0.93, p=0.011). [12] Cardiac function is not worsened by exercise training. In fact, a small but significant improvement of ejection fraction and reduction in cardiomegaly was observed in one prospective randomized trial. [13] In a recent multicenter randomized controlled trial of 2331 stable heart failure patients, a non-significant reduction was seen for mortality (189 [16%] in the exercise training group vs 198 [17%] in the usual care group; HR 0.96 [95% CI, 0.79-1.17];p=.70). There was a tendency towards a significant reduction in cardiovascular mortality or cardiovascular hospitalization (632 [55%] vs 677 [58%]; HR 0.92 [95% CI, 0.83-1.03];p=.14), and cardiovascular mortality or heart failure hospitalization (344 [30%] vs 393 [34%]; HR 0.87 [95% CI, 0.75-1.00];p=.06). After adjustment for highly prognostic baseline characteristics, exercise training was associated with modest significant reductions for both all-cause mortality or hospitalization and cardiovascular mortality or heart failure hospitalization. [14] Exercise training conferred modest but statistically significant improvements in self-reported health status compared with usual care without training. Improvements occurred early (3 months) and persisted over time (2.5 years). [15]

In a systematic review, Smart et al. found no reports of deaths that were directly related to exercise during more than 60 000 PTH in patients with heart failure. [9]

Patients with an ICD often have chronic heart failure or ischemic heart disease and would therefore profit from cardiac rehabilitation. In a study of 92 ICD-patients, training effects were smaller for peak $V0_2$ (mL/min/kg) in the ICD group than in the control group (+18% vs. +27%; p= 0.006). Five appropriate and one inappropriate shock were delivered during training (3478 PTH). [16] Studies evaluating the benefit of psychological counselling are ongoing.

Heart transplantation patients are usually strongly deconditioned. The transplanted heart also has an altered response to exercise due to denervation. [17] There is growing clinical consensus that specific endurance and resistance training regimens in heart transplant patients can be efficacious adjunctive therapies in the prevention of immunosuppression-induced adverse effects and the reversal of pathophysiological consequences associated with cardiac denervation and antecedent heart failure. [18,19]

Overall, in rehabilitation settings under supervision, rates of adverse events during exercise have consistently been low. In a study of 1909 patients referred to our cardiac rehabilitation programme in UZ Leuven from 1979 to 2000, improvements in peak $V0_2$ and exercise duration averaged 26%. The intake of anti-arrhythmics (OR 5.5; $p<0.001$) and the presence of ST-segment depression at baseline exercise testing (OR = 1.6: $p<0.001$) were predictive for serious complications. The occurrence of events requiring resuscitation was higher at the sports club (Phase III rehabilitation) than at the ambulatory, supervised in–hospital exercise programme (Phase II rehabilitation), confirming the data from Franklin et al. [20] In this study from 1982 to 1998, rates of major cardiovascular events range from 1 per 49 315 (Phase II) to 1 per 58 451 (Phase II and III combined) PTH, with only 2 cardiac arrests per 292 254 PTH, both successfully resuscitated. [21]

The SIGN (Scottish Intercollegiate Guidelines Network) recommend staff with basic life support training and the ability to use a defibrillator for low to moderate risk patients, and the immediate access to a hospital emergency team and advanced life support facilities for high risk patients or classes offering high intensity exercise. [22]

Program Components of Cardiac Rehabilitation

Cardiac rehabilitation is conventionally divided into three phases:

- Phase 1: acute/subacute rehabilitation: in-hospital mobilization, education and psychosocial counselling/referral (first days or weeks after admission)
- Phase 2: convalescence: reconditioning/early lifestyle modification
- Phase 3: long-term maintenance program

We will focus on the second phase, after the patient is discharged from the hospital and been referred for participation in the cardiac rehabilitation program.

1) First visit: Medical evaluation

1. History
- Medical history
- Drug therapy
- Occupational status
- Physical activity, identification of barriers
- Diet
- Smoking status, readiness to quit
- Psychosocial problems such as denial, depression, anxiety, social isolation, anger and hostility by means of an interview, standardized questionnaire or both
- Lipid, glycemic and blood pressure control

2. Physical examination, including blood pressure, height, weight, waist circumference
3. Electrocardiogram at rest
4. Exercise test

Assessment of exercise capacity in the clinical context

5. Determine level of risk

The SIGN (Scottish Ilegiate Guidelines Network) guideline on Cardiac Rehabilitation 2002 states that for most patients clinical risk stratification for assessment of suitability for exercise can be based on history, examination, resting ECG combined with a functional capacity test. [22]

2) Exercise therapy in cardiovascular diseases

Physical exercise has developed over the last two decades from rehabilitation in the 'restorement' sense to exercise treatment of cardio-vascular diseases as an evidence-based and guideline-orientated treatment option to improve prognosis.

Endurance training is known to improve maximal oxygen uptake, to induce cardiovascular adaptations, to improve cardiovascular risk factors and to burn calories resulting in weight loss. Resistance training on the other hand, is known to improve muscular strength, muscular strength endurance and to enhance muscle mass. It has an additive function in augmenting the basal metabolism, resulting in improved weight loss. It improves independency and reduces falling tendency in the elderly. [23]

Three to four aerobic moderate-intensity endurance exercise training sessions per week, with a duration of 30 to 40 minutes each, are recommended in patients with CAD. Moderate intensity can be defined by a training heart rate of 64-76% of the maximal heart rate, or at an intensity of 45-67% of the maximal oxygen uptake, or at an intensity of 40-59% of the heart rate reserve or oxygen uptake reserve. [24]

Resistance training exercise is recommended for implementation in primary and secondary cardiovascular disease-prevention programs. Moderate intensity programmes (10 repetitions) involving mostly dynamic stress are usually recommended for cardiac patients.

Interval training seems to be more effective as compared to continuous aerobic exercise training to improve maximal oxygen uptake. Peripheral musculature is trained more intensively by short intervals at higher intensity, whereas cardiovascular load is not higher than in continuous aerobic exercise. Especially weak patients with very limited exercise capacity might profit from interval training to improve performance of daily life activities.

3) Education and counselling

Patient education on heart disease

Education enables patients to manage their illness, to adopt and maintain healthy lifestyles and improves adherence to medications. [25] Education programs have demonstrated a measurable impact on blood pressure, exercise, diet and mortality. [26]

Dietary Counselling

Dietary counselling should focus on two goals: there is often the need for weight reduction, necessitating calorie restriction and on the other hand there's the need for a healthy food intake.

Reduced-calorie diets by a deficit of 750 kcal per day from baseline, result in a mean weight loss of approximately 6 kg after 6 months, regardless of whether it emphasizes protein, fat or carbohydrates. [27]

In the early 1950s, the classic diet-heart hypothesis was developed, postulating dietary saturated fat and cholesterol as causative factors in the development of atherosclerosis. [28] The diet-heart hypothesis resulted in the advice of healthy eating according to the food pyramid, with adjustments for the quantity and quality of fatty acids and cholesterol: energy distribution is recommended to be 30% from fat, with 7% of saturated fat, 20% of mono unsaturated fat and 10% of poly unsaturated fat, 55% from carbohydrates and 15% from protein. Trans fatty acids e.g. should be avoided Subjects eating diets emphasizing on fruits, vegetables, cereals, potatoes, beans, nuts, seeds, olive oil, low-fat dairy products, fish and poultry as in the Mediterranean diet, have a 50 to 70% lower risk of recurrent heart disease. [30] Intake of fish oil supplements (omega 3 fatty acids) after myocardial infarction decreases the risk of death by 14 to 20% and the risk of cardiovascular death by 17 to 30% after 3.5 years. [30] Increasing fibre intake or taking antioxidants such as β-carotene, vitamin E, vitamin C, selenium or multivitamin supplements has shown no benefit in reducing the risk of CAD, after adjusting for CAD risk factors. [30,31]

Smoking Cessation

Smoking cessation reduces the risk of subsequent mortality and further cardiac events among patients with coronary artery disease by 50%. [32] Smoking cessation therefore should be the primary objective of treatment for people with coronary artery disease. The aim is a complete cessation of smoking. Smoking cessation counselling interventions should begin during the hospitalisation period and should include at least one month of follow-up supportive contact after discharge. Less than 1-2% of heavily dependent smokers achieve this goal through will-power alone. The outcome improves with individual counselling, group therapy, psychological and pharmacological support. Acupuncture, hypnosis and relaxation have no demonstrated efficacy on smoking cessation, whereas self-help material may offer a small benefit. [33]

Pharmacotherapy should be part of the in-hospital intervention in addition to counselling when clinically indicated. [34]

Nicotine replacement therapy (NRT) is proven to be safe in patients with heart disease and increases the probability of successful cessation by 50 to 70%, independent of the intensity of additional support provided to the individual. The chance of being abstinent from smoking for any form of NRT relative to control (placebo) was 1.58 (risk ratio; 95%CI 1.50-1.65). [35]

A meta-analysis shows that bupropion nearly doubles cessation rates with an OR of 1.94 (95% CI 1.72-2.19), an increased efficacy compared to NRT. [36] For smokers starting bupropion therapy, a target quitting date should be set for 2 weeks after the initiation of treatment. Therapy starts with a dose of 150 mg once daily for 6 days, followed by the target dose of 150 mg twice daily for 7 to 9 weeks, after which tapering of dose is required until stopped.

Randomized controlled trials demonstrated that varenicline has superior efficacy compared with placebo and bupropion. The pooled OR for validated continous abstinence at 12 months for varenicline versus placebo was 3.22 (95% CI 2.43-4.27) and 1.66 (95% CI 1.28-2.16) for varenicline versus bupropion. [37]

Varenicline can be prescribed safely in patients with heart disease. For smokers starting varenicline therapy, a target quitting date should be set for 1 week after the initiation of treatment. Varenicline treatment should be initiated with a 1-week dose-adjustment period, to reduce nausea. Therapy starts with a dose of 0.5 mg once daily on days 1 through 3, 0.5 mg twice daily on days 4 through 7, and the target dose of 1.0 mg twice daily starting on day 8 (i.e., the target quitting date). In patients with severe renal impairment (estimated creatinine clearance < 30 ml/min), a reduction in the dose to 0.5 mg daily is recommended. Therapy may be discontinued abruptly after 12 to 24 weeks, with no tapering required. [33]

A recent randomized clinical trial compared cessation rates among smokers who receive pharmacotherapy alone (n = 250) or supplemented with either 2 counseling calls (n = 249; moderate-intensity disease management) or up to 6 counseling calls (n = 251; high-intensity disease management) every 6 months. Pharmacotherapy consisted of a 6-week course of a nicotine patch (21 mg/d) or a 7-week course of sustained-release bupropion (150 mg twice daily). The self-reported abstinence at 24 months was 27.9% and 23.5% in the high-intensity and moderate-intensity disease management groups respectively (OR, 1.33;CI 0.88-2.02). Secondary overall analyses (0 to 24 months), showed that self-reported abstinence rates were higher in the combined disease management groups than in the pharmacotherapy-alone group (OR 1.47; CI 1.08-2.00). [38]

Psychological Risk Factors and Behavioural Support

Depression

In a study from 1988, just less than 20% of the patients suffering from CAD met the criteria for major depression. This depressed group turned out to be about 2 to 3 times more likely to develop a serious adverse cardiac complication over the next 12 months.[39] Several other investigators studying post-myocardial infarction patients have also found a higher mortality with e.g. a hazard ratio of 4.29 (95% CI 3.14-5.44,P=0.013) associated with depression. [40]

Cardiovascular risk factors might contribute to a certain extent for this association, but it is likely that pathophysiological mechanisms, such as changes in the autonomic nervous system, neuroendocrine and platelet activation and endothelial dysfunction that are seen in depression account for a substantial portion of the increased cardiovascular death rate. [41]

Treatment with tricyclic antidepressants is too risky in cardiac patients. [42] Evidence has accumulated that selective serotonine reuptake inhibitors antidepressants are safe and effective and there is a suggestion that they reduce not only depression but medical adverse events as well, with the greatest benefit in the recurrently and severely depressed subpopulations. [43] However, that evidence is not definitive and the reason behind the association between depression and cardiovascular morbidity and mortality remains uncertain. [44]

A systematic overview published by our group, provides a step-by-step guide in order to help non-psychiatric healthcare providers in dealing with depressed patients. [45]

Anxiety

Anxiety disorders are linked to the development of cardiac events in the general population, with the excess mortality being confined to sudden cardiac death in previously healthy subjects (relative risk among men scoring 3 or higher on the phobia index was 6.08; 95% CI 2.35-15.73). [46]

In a study of Strik et al. in 318 men after a first myocardial infarction, symptoms of both depression (HR 2.32, 95% CI 1.04-5.18, p=0.039) and anxiety (HR 3.01, 95% CI 1.20-7.60, p= 0.019) were associated with fatal and non-fatal myocardial infarction. [47] Also in-hospital cardiac complications after myocardial infarction, such as recurrent ischemia, reinfarction, congestive heart failure, and ventricular arrhythmia requiring intervention, are increased by post-MI anxiety as an independent predictor (OR 1.17; P=.015, 95% CI=1.03–1.32). [48]

There are several potential mechanisms by which post-MI anxiety could lead to cardiac complications in the post-MI period. First, acute anxiety and stress are associated with increased sympathetic nervous system activity. [49] In addition, anxiety is associated with increased platelet aggregation in response to catecholamines. [50]

Regarding health care consumption, anxiety (OR 2.00, 95% CI 1.24-3.22, p= 0.005), but not depression or hostility, was a predictor of cardiac rehospitalisation and frequent visits at the cardiac outpatient clinic. A subset of anxious patients may experience noncardiac chest pain, which may be induced or exacerbated by anxiety. [51]

These data suggest that screening for and treatment of anxiety in the post-MI setting could be useful to prevent cardiac complications, but further treatment studies are needed to determine the impact of anxiety treatment on post-MI in-hospital cardiac outcomes. [52]

Personality Factors, Character Traits

Type A individuals are characterised by their wish to do too much in too little time, competitiveness, frustration, and aggression. Prospective studies of general population samples have found that the pattern, and more specifically hostility and anger, are associated with increased risk of CHD. [53]

In a study of 303 patients with CAD, type-D personality, i.e. the tendency to suppress emotional distress, was an independent predictor for both cardiac and noncardiac mortality. Rate of death was 27% for type-D patients versus 7% for patients without type-D ($p<0.00001$) at follow-up after 6 to 10 years. [54]

In another study, evaluating psychological traits in 246 patients at discharge of an acute myocardial infarction, low emotional sensitivity, i.e. an inability to express emotion and adapting to society or coping, and insecurity were predictive of cardiac death at 8-year follow-up (relative risk 4.18; p=0.003). [55]

On the other hand, in a large cohort study the personality trait of permissiveness/low self-confidence may be protective against non-fatal myocardial infarction, particularly in women (relative risk 0.59 [95% CI 0.40–0.85]). [56]

Life stress

Emotional stress may precipitate cardiac events in people who are predisposed to such events. On the day of the earthquake in Los Angeles 1994, there was a sharp increase in the number of sudden deaths from cardiac causes that were related to atherosclerotic cardiovascular disease, from a daily average (±SD) of 4.6±2.1 in the preceding week to 24 on the day of the earthquake ($z=4.41$, $p<0.001$). During the six days after the earthquake, the number of sudden deaths declined to below the baseline value, to an average of 2.7±1.2 per day. [57] In a more recent study, the effects of the terrorist attacks of 9/11 on cardiovascular outcomes are evaluated over 3 years. Acute stress responses to the 9/11 attacks were associated with a 53% increased incidence of cardiovascular ailments over the 3 subsequent years, even after adjusting for multiple risk factors. Among individuals reporting ongoing worry about terrorism post-9/11, high 9/11-related acute stress symptoms predicted increased risk of physician-diagnosed heart problems 2 to 3 years following the attacks (rate ratios, 4.67 at 2 years and 3.22 at 3 years). [58]

Social Isolation

Emotional support was measured in a study of Berkman et al., by responses to the following question: "Can you count on anyone to provide you with emotional support (talking over problems or helping you make a difficult decision)?" The sources of support were counted (0, 1 or ≥2). The lack of emotional support, assessed before myocardial infarction, is independently related to risk for death in the subsequent 6 months. Seventy six of 194 patients (39%) died in the first 6 months after myocardial infarction. In multiple logistic regression analyses, lack of emotional support was significantly associated with 6-month mortality (odds ratio, 2.9; 95% CI, 1.2-6.9) after controlling for severity of myocardial infarction, comorbidity, risk factors such as smoking and hypertension, and sociodemographic factors. [59]

Low levels of social and economic resources identify an important high-risk group among medically treated patients with coronary artery disease, independent of important medical prognostic factors. In a study in 1965 patients with CAD, patients with annual household incomes of $ 40,000 or more had an unadjusted 5-year survival of 91%, compared with 76% in patients with incomes of $10,000 or less (Cox model adjusted hazard ratio, 1.9; 95% CI 1.57-2.32; p=.002). Similarly, unmarried patients without a confidant had an unadjusted 5-year survival rate of 50%, compared with 82% in patients who were married, had a confidant or both (adjusted hazard ratio, 3.34; 95% CI 1.84-6.20; p<.0001). [60]

Sexual Problems

Sexual dysfunction is highly prevalent in patients with cardiovascular disease of both sexes and adversely affects patients' quality of life and well-being. [61] Erectile dysfunction is reported in up to 68.3% of patients with hypertension and in 40% of patients with coronary artery disease. It mostly is due to the vascular disease itself, but it may also be secondary to or aggravated by the intake of diuretics, beta-blockers and centrally acting sympatholytic antihypertensive drugs. Dose reduction or the newer beta-blocker nebivolol might solve the problem. Other agents such as calcium antagonists or angiotensive-converting enzyme inhibitors seem to be of little influence, whereas angiotensin II receptor (AT1) blockers might have beneficial effects on sexual function. [62,63] Sildenafil and vardenafil can be used safely in cardiac patients, although serious adverse events, especially significant hypotension, can occur and therefore co-administration with nitrates is absolutely contra-indicated.

Vocational Counselling

Return to work is one of the important goals of rehabilitation of patients with heart disease. Despite the well-documented effects of cardiac rehabilitation on functional capacity and psychological well-being, there is contradicting evidence regarding whether rehabilitation programmes can influence this return. Vocational rehabilitation as part of cardiac rehabilitation is to evaluate whether returning to work is safe and realistic, and to assist patients to resume or maintain work.

Successful return to work reduces the financial burden of disease for the patient and society. It is estimated that up to 80% of patients with uncomplicated myocardial infarction will return to work. The time for returning to work has decreased from 4 months after an event in 1970 to approximately 2 months in 1990. However, many patients do not resume work. Predictors of difficulties to resume work are increased age, low socio-economic status, job characteristics, negative expectations concerning return to work and level of depression and anxiety. In 2500 randomly selected CABG-patients, employment fell from 56% in the year prior to CABG to 42% in the year after. Workers in 'blue collar' occupations were more likely to reduce their work status than those in 'white collar' occupations (46% versus 29%, $p < 0.001$). Independent predictors of reducing employment were increasing age (9% per year, 99% CI:1.6-1.11, $p < 0.001$), 'blue collar' versus 'white collar' occupation (OR: 2.1, 99% CI: 1.4-3.1) and female sex (OR: 2.1, 99% CI: 1.1-3.6). Health-related quality of life score among patients younger than 60 was better for those who returned to work after CABG. [64]

Early identification of patients who are at risk of prolonged absence due to physical or psychological reasons is important. The job characteristics, legal and security demands, as well as physical and psychological demands of the job need to be addressed. Intervention can consist of psychological support, adaptation of the exercise programme for special needs at work and, if necessary, help in searching a new adapted job.

4) Medical evaluation during/at the end of cardiac rehabilitation

In the long term, most people with cardiac disease receive most or all of their care in primary care. Once the process of short term recovery is complete, the emphasis of cardiac rehabilitation shifts to long term maintenance of physical activity and lifestyle change, with appropriate secondary prophylactic drug therapy.

The cardiac rehabilitation specialist will re-evaluate the patient for clinical status, risk factors and cardiac medication. The boundaries between cardiac rehabilitation, secondary prevention and normal medical care are blurred and the overall aim is comprehensive cardiac care. Good communication is primordial. In particular, tailored information should be provided with details of treatment and cardiac rehabililtation to date, ongoing monitoring required and future treatment planned.

A final maximal exercise test, preferably an ergospirometry, is performed. A final multidisciplinary report including change in clinical status (symptoms, body weight, blood pressure etc.), control of cardiac and psychosocial risk factors (social support, depression, anxiety etc.) and attention points for the future will be communicated to the referring cardiologist and general practitioner. [65]

References

[1] WHO Committee. Rehabilitation after cardiovascular diseases, with special emphasis on developing countries: a report of a WHO Committee. *World Health Organ Tech Rep Ser*, 1993, 831, 1-122.

[2] Committee on Exercise and Cardiac Rehabilitation of the Council on Clinical Cardiology. Core components of cardiac rehabilitation/ secondary prevention programs. A statement for health professionals by the Committee on Exercise and Cardiac Rehabilitation of the Council on Clinical Cardiology. *Circulation*, 2000, 102, 1069-1073.

[3] Wenger NK, Froelicher ES, Smith LK et al. Cardiac rehabilitation. Clinical Practice Guideline No. 17, AHCPR Publication No.96-0672. Rockville, MD: US Department of Health and Human Services, Public Health Service, Agency for Health Care Policy and Research, and the *National Heart Lung and Blood Institute*, 1995.

[4] Hambrecht R, Walther C, Möbius-Winkler S, Gielen S, Linke A, conradi K, Erbs S, Kluge R, Kendziorra K, Sabri O, Sick P, Schuler G. Percutaneous coronary angioplasty compared with exercise training in patients with stable coronary artery disease – a randomised trial. *Circulation*, 2004, 109, 1371-8.

[5] Taylor, RS; Brown, A; Ebrahim, S; Lolliffe, J; Noorani, H; Rees, K; et al. Exercise-based rehabilitation for patients with coronary heart disease: systematic review and meta-analysis of randomized controlled trials. *Am J Med*, 2004, 116, 682-692.

[6] Haskell, WL. Cardiovascular complications during exercise training of cardiac patients. *Circulation*, 1978, 57, 920-924.

[7] Van Camp, SP; Peterson, RA. Cardiovascular complication of out-patient cardiac rehabilitation programs. *JAMA*, 1986, 256, 1160-1163.

[8] Coats, AJ; Adamopoulos, S; Meyer, TE; Conway, J; Sleight, P. Effects of physical training in chronic heart failure. *Lancet*, 1990, 335, 63-65.

[9] Smart, N; Marwick, TH. Exercise training for patients with heart failure: a systematic review of factors that improve mortality and morbidity. *Am J Med*, 2004, 116, 693-706.

[10] Rees, K; Taylor, RS; Singh, S; Coats, AJS; Ebrahim, S. Exercise based rehabilitation for heart failure. Cochrane Database of Systematic reviews 2004;Issue 3. Art. No.: CD003331.DOI: 10.1002/14651858. CD003331. pub2.

[11] Austin, J; Williams, WR; Ross, L; Hutchison, S. Five-year follow-up findings from a randomized controlled trial of cardiac rehabilitation for heart failure. *Eur J Cardiovasc Prev Rehabil*, 2008, 15(2), 162-7.

[12] Piepoli, MF; Davos, C; Francis, DP; Coats, AJ. Exercise training meta-analysis of trials in patients with chronic heart failure (ExTraMATCH). *Br Med J*, 2004, 328, 189.

[13] Hambrecht, R; Gielen, S; Linke, A; Fiehn, E; Yu, J; Walther, C; et al. Effects of exercise training on left-ventricular function and peripheral resistance in patients with chronic heart failure. A randomized trial. *JAMA*, 2000, 283, 3095-3101.

[14] O'Connor, CM; Whellan, DJ; Lee, KL; Keteyian, SJ; Cooper, LS; Eklis, SJ; Leifer, ES; Kraus, WE; Kitzman, DW; Blumenthal, JA; Rendall, DS; Miller, NH; Fleg, JL; Schulman, KA; McKelvie, RS; Zannad, F; Piña, IL. for the HF-ACTION Investigators. Efficacy and safety of exercise training in patients with chronic heart failure. HF-ACTION randomized controlled trial. *JAMA*, 2009, 301(14), 1439-1450.

[15] Flynn, KE; Piña, LI; Whellan, DJ; Lin, L; Blumenthal, JA; Ellis, JS; Fine, JL; Howlett, J; Keteyian, SJ; Kitzman, DW; Kraus, WE; Miller, NH; Schulman, KA; Spertus, JA; 0'Connor, CM; Weinfurt, KP. Effects of exercise training on health status in patients with chronic heart failure. HF-ACTION randomized controlled trial. *JAMA*, 2009, 301(14), 1451-1459.

[16] Vanhees, L; Kornaat, M; Defoor, J; Aufdemkampe, G; Schepers, D; Stevens, A; van Exel, H; van den Beld, J; Heidbuchel, H; Fagard, R. Effect of exercise training in patients with an implantable cardioverter defibrillator. *Eur Heart J*, 2004, 25, 1120-6.

[17] Scot, JM; Esch, BT; Hayckowsky, MJ; Warburton, DE; Toma, M; Jelani, A; Taylor, D; Paterson, I; Poppe, D; Liang Y; Thompson, R.

Cardiovascular responses to incremental and sustained submaximal exercise in heart transplant recipients. *Am J Physiol Heart Circ Physiol*, 2009, 296, H350-H358.

[18] Braith, RW; Edwards, DG. Exercise following heart transplantation. *Sports Med*, 2000, 30(3), 171-92.

[19] Pokan, R; VonDuvillard, SP; Ludwig, J; Rohrer, A; Hofmann, P; Wonisch, M; Gerhard, S; Schmid, P; Pacher, R; Bachl, N. Effect of high-volume and –intensity endurance training in heart transplant recipients. *Med Sci Sports Exerc*, 2004, 36, 2011-2016.

[20] Vanhees, L; Stevens, A; Schepers, D; Defoor, J; Rademakers, F; Fagard, R. Determinants of the effects of physical training and of the complications requiring resuscitation during exercise in patients with cardiovascular disease. *Eur J Cardiovasc Prev Rehabil*, 2004, 11, 304-312.

[21] Franklin, BA; Bonzheim, K; Gordon, S; Timmis, GC. Safety of medically supervised outpatient cardiac rehabilitation exercise therapy: a 16-year follow-up. *Chest*, 1998, 114(3), 902-6.

[22] Cardiac Rehabilitation. A national clinical guideline. Scottish Intercollegiate Guidelines Network 2002. Available from: http://www.sign.ac.uk/pdf/sign57.pdf

[23] Pollock, ML; Franklin, BA; Balady, GJ; Chaitman, BL; Fleg, JL; Fletcher, B; Limacher, M; Piña, IL; Stein, RA; Williams, M; Bazzarre, T. Resistance exercise in individuals with and without cardiovascular disease: benefits, rationale, safety, and prescription, Council on Clinical Cardiology, American Heart Association. *Circulation*, 2000, 101, 828-833.

[24] Howley, ET. Type of activity: resistance, aerobic and leisure versus occupational physical activity. *Med Sci Sports Exerc*, 2001, 33(6), S364-9.

[25] Mullen, PD; Mains, DA; Velez, R. A meta-analysis of controlled trials of cardiac patient education. *Patient Educ Couns*, 1992, 19, 143.

[26] Ornish, D; Brown, SE; Scherwitz, LW; Billings, JH; Armstrong, WT; Ports, TA; et al. Can lifestyle changes reverse coronary heart disease? The Lifestyle Heart Trail. *Lancet*, 1990, 336, 129-133.

[27] Sacks, FM; Bray, GA; Carey, VJ; Smith, SR; Ryan, DH; Anton, SD; McManus, K; Champagne, CM; Bishop, LM; Laranjo, N; Leboff, MS; Rood, JC; de Jonge, L; Greenway, FL; Loria, CM; Obarzanek, E;

Williamson, DA. Comparison of weight-loss diets with different compositions of fat, protein, and carbohydrates. *NEJM*, 2009, 360(9), 923-5.

[28] Gordon, T. The diet-heart idea. Outline of a history. Am J Epidemiol 1988, 127, 220-225.

[29] De Lorgeril, M; Salen, P; Martin, JL; Monjaud, I; Delaye, J; Mamelle, N. Mediterranean diet, traditional risk factors, and the rate of cardiovascular complications after myocardial infarction: final report of the Lyon Diet Heart Study. *Circulation*, 1999, 99, 779-785.

[30] Dietary supplementation with n-3 polyunsaturated fatty acids and vitamin E after myocardial infarction: results of the GISSI-Prevenzione trial. Gruppo Italiano per lo Studio della Sopravvivenza nell'Infarto miocardico. *Lancet*, 1999, 354, 447-455.

[31] Wolk, A; Manson, JE; Stampfer, MJ; Coldity, GA; Hu, FB; Speizer, FE et al. Long-term intake of dietary fiber and decreased risk of coronary heart disease among women. *JAMA*, 1999, 281, 1998-2004.

[32] Wilhelmsson, C; Vedin, JA; Elmfeldt, D; Tibblin, G; Wilhelmsen, L. Smoking and myocardial infarction. Lancet, 1975, 1, 415-420.

[33] Stead, LF; Lancaster, T. Group behaviour therapy programmes for smoking cessation (review). The Cochrane Collaboration. *Cochrane Database Syst Rev.*, 2005, (2), CD001007.

[34] Rigotti, N; Munafo, MR; Stead, LF. Interventions for smoking cessation in hospitalized patients (review).The Cochrane Collaboration. Cochrane Database Syst Rev., 2007, (3), CD001837.

[35] Stead, LF; Perera, R; Bullen, C; Mant, D; Lancaster, T. Nicotine replacement therapy for smoking cessation. *Cochrane Database of Systematic Reviews*, 2008, Issue 1. Art. No.:CD000146. DOI:10.1002/14651858. CD000146.pub3.

[36] Hughes, JR; Stead, LF; Lancaster T. *Cochrane Database Syst Rev.*, 2007, 1, CD00031.

[37] Gonzales, D; Rennard, SI; Nides, M; et al. Varenicline, an α4β2 nicotinic acetylcholine receptor partial agonist, vs sustained-release bupropion and placebo for smoking cessation. A randomized controlled trial. *JAMA*, 2006, 296, 47-55.

[38] Ellerbeck, EF; Mahnken, JD; Cupertino, AP; Cox, LS; Greiner, KA; Mussulman, LM; Nazir, N; Shireman, TI; Resnicow, K; Ahluwalia, JS.

Effect of varying levels of disease management on smoking cessation. A randomized trial. *Ann Intern Med*, 2009, 150, 437-446.
[39] Carney, RM; Rich, MW; Freedland, DE; Saini, J; Tevelde, A; Simeone, C; Clark, K. Major depressive disorder predicts cardiac events in patients with coronary artery disease. *Psychosom Med*, 1988, 50, 627-633.
[40] Frasure-Smith, N; Lesperance, F; Talajic, M. Depression following myocardial infarction: impact on 6-month survival *JAMA*, 1993, 270, 1819-1825.
[41] Glassman, AH; Shapiro, PA. Depression and the course of coronary artery disease. *Am J Psychiatry*, 1998, 155, 4-11.
[42] Glassman, AH; Roose, SP; Bigger, JT. Jr: The safety of tricyclic antidepressants in cardiac patients: risk/benefit reconsidered. JAMA 1993, 269, 2673-2675.
[43] Regan, KL. Depression treatment with selective serotonin reuptake inhibitors for the postacute coronary syndrome population: a literature review. *J Cardiovasc Nurs*, 2008, 23(6), 489-96.
[44] Glassman, A. Depression and cardiovascular disease. Pharmacopsychiatry, 2008, 41(6), 221-5.
[45] Dobbels, F; De Geest, S; Vanhees, L; Schepens, K; Fagard, R; Vanhaecke, J. Depression and the heart: a systematic overview of definition, measurement, consequences and treatment of depression in cardiovascular disease. *Eur J Carciovasc Nurs*, 2002, 1(1), 45-55.
[46] Kawachi, I; Colditz, GA; Ascherio, A; Rimm, EB; Giovannucci, E; Stampfer, MJ; et al. Prospective study of phobic anxiety and risk of coronary heart disease in men. *Circulation*, 1994, 89, 1992-1997.
[47] Strik, JJ; Denollet, J; Lousberg, R; Honig, A. Comparing symptoms of depression and anxiety as predictors of cardiac events and increased health care consumption after myocardial infarction. *J Am Coll Cardiol*, 2003, 42, 1801-7.
[48] Huffman, JC; Smith, FA; Blais, MA; Januzzi, JL; Fricchione, GL. Anxiety, independent of depressive symptoms, is associated with in-hospital cardiac complications after acute myocardial infarction. *J Psychosom Res*, 2008, 65, 557-563.
[49] Rozanski, A; Blumenthal, JA; Kaplan, J. Impact of psychological factors on the pathogenesis of cardiovascular disease and implications for therapy. Circulation, 1999, 99, 2192-217.

[50] Simpson, MT; Olewine, DA; Jenkins, CD; et al. Exercise-induced catecholamines and platelet aggregation in the coronary-prone behaviour pattern. *Psychosom Med*, 1974, 36, 476-87.

[51] Logue, MB; Thomas, AM; Barbee, JG; Hoehn-Saric, R; Maddock, RJ; Schwab, J; Smith, RD; Sullivan, M; Beitman, BD. Generalized anxiety disorder patients seek evaluation for cardiological symptoms at the same rate as patients with panic disorder. *J Psychiatr Res*, 1993, 27, 55-9.

[52] Wheatley, D. Anxiolytic drug use in cardiovascular disease: an overview. *Psychopharmacol Bull*, 1984, 20, 649-59.

[53] Haynes, SG; Feinleib, M; Kannel, WB. The relationship of psychosocial factors to coronary heart disease in the Framingham study: III, eight-year incidence of coronary heart disease. Am J Epidemiol 1980;111:37-58.

[54] Denollet, J; Sys, SU; Stroobant, N; Rombouts, H; Gillebert, TC; Brusaert, DL. Personality as independent predictor of long term mortality in patients with coronary heart disease. *Lancet*, 1996, 347(8999), 417-421.

[55] Carpeggiani, C; Emdin, M; Bonaguidi, F; Landi, P; Michelassi, C; Trivella, MG; Macerata, A; L'Abbate, A. Personality traits and heart rate variability predict long-term cardiac mortality after myocardial infarction. *Eur Heart J*, 2005, 26, 1612-1617.

[56] Whiteman, MC; Deary, IJ; Lee, AJ; Fowkes, FGR. Submissiveness and protection from coronary heart disease in the general population: Edinburgh Artery Study. *Lancet*, 1997, 350, 541-45.

[57] Leor, J; Poole, WK; Kloner, RA. Sudden cardiac death triggered by an earthquake. *N Engl J Med*, 1996, 334, 413-419.

[58] Holman, EA; Cohen Silver, R; Poulin, M; et al. Terrorism, acute stress, and cardiovascular health. A 3-year national study following the September 11th attacks. *Arch Gen Psychiatry*, 2008, 65, 73-80.

[59] Berkman, LF; Leo-Summers, L; Horwitz, RI. Emotional support and survival after myocardial infarction. A prospective, population-based study of the elderly. *Ann Intern Med*, 1992, 117, 1003-1009.

[60] Williams, RB; Barefoot, JC; Califf, RM; Haney, TL; Saunders, WB; Pryor, DB; et al. Prognostic importance of social and economic resources among medically treated patients with angiographically documented coronary artery disease. *JAMA*, 1992, 267, 520-524.

[61] DeBusk, R; Drory, Y; Goldstein, I; Jackson, G; Kaul, S; Kimmel, SE; et al. Management of sexual dysfunction in patients with cardiovascular disease: recommendations of The Princeton Consensus Panel. *Am J Cardiol*, 2000, 86, 175-181.

[62] Barksdale, JD; Gardner, SF. The impact of first-line antihypertensive drugs on erectile dysfunction. *Pharmacotherapy*, 1999, 19, 573-581.

[63] Manolis, A; Doumas, M. Sexual dysfunction: the 'prima ballerina' of hypertension-related quality-of-life complications. *J Hypertens*, 2008, 26(11), 2074-84.

[64] Bradhaw, PJ; Jamrozik, K; Gilfillan, IS; Thompson, PL. Return to work after coronary artery bypass grafting in a population of long term survivors. *Heart Lung and Circulation*, 2005, 14(3), 191-16.

[65] Dendale, P; Dereppe, H; De Sutter, J; Laruelle, C; Vaes, J; Lamotte, M; Deroeck, A; Mallefroy, M; Heyndrickx, B; Berger, J; Kostucki, W; Fortuin, A; Hansen, D; Brohet, C; Vanhees, L. Position paper of the Belgian Working Group on Cardiovascular Prevention and Rehabilitation: cardiovascular rehabilitation. *Acta Cardiologica*, 2008, 63(6), 673-681.

In: Cardiac Rehabilitaiton
Editor: J. T. Halliday, pp. 143-163
ISBN: 978-1-60741-918-1

Chapter VI

Metabolic Syndrome, Myocardial Aging, and Diastolic Heart Failure: Related Mechanisms and Implications for Cardiac Rehabilitation

***Eduardo Borges de Oliveira*[1], *Jarbas S. Roriz-Filho*[1], *Idiane Rosset*[2] *and Matheus Roriz-Cruz*[3]**
[1]Division of Geriatrics. Department of Internal Medicine. School of Medicine of Ribeirão Preto at University of São Paulo-RP, Brazil
[2]Division of Gerontological Nursing. Faculty of Nursing. Brazilian Federal University of Rio Grande do Sul State, Brazil
[3]Division of Geriatric Medicine. Department of Internal Medicine. Brazilian Federal University of Rio Grande do Sul State, Brazil

Abstract

Metabolic Syndrome (Met.S) consists of a cluster of symptoms including abdominal obesity, glucose intolerance, low HDL-cholesterol, high triglycerides, and high blood pressure. All of these components seem to be caused, at least partially, by the same pathophysiologic process, named Insulin Resistance (IR). IR has been recognized as having a central role in regulating biological aging. Hyperglycemia and hyperinsulinism are two consequences of IR, both of which being associated with an increased formation of Reactive Oxygen Species (ROS) and Advance Glucose Endproducts (AGEs). ROS and AGE are the key points for each of the two main theories of aging: oxidative stress and protein glycation, respectively. IR is, in fact, a mechanism intrinsically associated with calorie ingestion; calorie restriction being the only proved way to extend life in mammals, including primates. Diabetic cardiomyopathy is well-known to be associated with myocardial aging and Diastolic Heart Failure (DHF). Evidences are accumulating that milder forms of IR and hyperglycemia are also associated with increased myocardial cell oxidative stress and protein glycation. Hyperinsulinism also causes capillary endothelial proliferation, contributing to microvascular ischemic myocardiopathy and, consequently, diastolic dysfunction. Hypertension, another component of Met.S, is the most common cause of (concentric) hypertrophic myocardiopathy, which can further impair ventricular complacence, contributing to DHF. Managing Met.S components in an integrated approach may contribute to cardiac rehabilitation in many ways. Losing weight by itself can ameliorate DHF by both direct and indirect mechanisms. Weight reduction would decrease the need for a continuously elevated cardiac output at rest which, by itself, would improve symptoms in heart failure. Adequately managing Met.S components may improve diastolic relaxation through two main mechanisms. First, tight control of blood pressure would prevent myocardial remodeling and even regress, to some degree, this process, improving diastolic function. Second, strict long-term glycemic control has the potential to decelerate myocardial aging and, additionally, improve diastolic function both by regressing cardiac microangiopathy and intracellular glucose utilization by the myocardial cell. Exercise is an essential part in the cardiac rehabilitation plan of the patient with IR-associated myocardiopathy. Independent of weight reduction, dynamic exercise is able to improve IR, diastolic function, and peripheral energy utilization, all mechanisms collaborating to rehabilitation on DHF.

1. Introduction

Metabolic Syndrome consists of a cluster of symptoms including abdominal obesity, glucose intolerance, low HDL-cholesterol, high triglycerides, and high blood pressure. All of these components seem to be caused, at least partially, be the same physiopathologic process, namely

Insulin Resistance (IR). IR has been recognized as having a central role in regulating biological aging.

Insulin regulates the uptake of glucose by the tissues and it storage as glucogen. The major sites of insulin action are the liver, fat tissue, skeletal muscle and the brain, and in special some regions with a high demand for glucose. Hyperglycemia and hyperinsulinism are two consequences of IR, both of which being associated with an increased formation of Reactive Oxygen Species (ROS) and Advance Glucose Endproducts (AGEs). ROS and AGE are the key points for each of the two main theories of aging: oxidative stress and protein glycation, respectively.

Diabetic cardiomyopathy is well-known to be associated with myocardial aging and Diastolic Heart Failure (DHF). Evidences are accumulating that milder forms of IR and hyperglycemia are also associated with increased myocardial cell oxidative stress and protein glycation. Hyperinsulinism also causes capillary endothelial proliferation, contributing to microvascular ischemic myocardiopathy and, consequently, diastolic dysfunction. Hypertension, another component of Metabolic Syndrome, is the most common cause of (concentric) hypertrophic myocardiopathy, which can further impair ventricular complacence, contributing to DHF.

In this chapter the authors will review: definitions, physiopathologic and clinical aspects of metabolic syndrome and myocardial aging; the relationships between them; their role in the physiopathology of diastolic heart failure; the importance of the right recognition and treatment of these entities for cardiac rehabilitation.

2. Definitions

2.1. Metabolic Syndrome

In 1988, Reaven noted that several risk factors commonly cluster together under one disorder entity that he originally described as syndrome X. This syndrome has been characterized by the co-occurrence of hypertension, some degree of glucose intolerance, high triglyceride levels and low high-density lipoprotein (HDL) concentrations. The basic abnormalities underlying syndrome X have been presented as the resistance of insulin to mediate glucose disposal. Due to this underlying pathophysiology, many authors have also used the term insulin resistance syndrome to define this aggregation of risk factors. The syndrome has also been given other names, including metabolic syndrome, plurimetabolic syndrome and 'deadly quartet'. More recently, the National Cholesterol Education Program's Adult Treatment Panel-III report (NCEP ATP-III) has recognized the importance of this syndrome in the prevention of cardiovascular disease (CVD). However, NCEP ATP-III, used the term metabolic syndrome for this clustering of metabolic risk factors. This term avoids the implication that insulin resistance is the primary or the only cause of associated risk factors. Since the description of the syndrome by Reaven[1], several other metabolic abnormalities have been associated with it, including obesity, particularly abdominal obesity, high apolipoprotein (apo) B levels, small dense low-density lipoprotein (LDL), and abnormalities in fibrinolysis and coagulation.

At least three different organizations have provided operational criteria in order to identify patients with the metabolic syndrome. However, these clinical criteria differ somewhat between these organizations. Tables 1, 2 and 3 summarize the criteria used by the NCEP ATP-III, the World Health Organization (WHO) and the American Association of Clinical Endocrinologists (AACE) to clinically identify the metabolic syndrome.

For NCEP ATP-III, when 3 out of the 5 characteristics listed in Table 1 are present, a diagnosis of metabolic syndrome can be made. It is the only guideline that considers waist circumference to express the level of adiposity. In the NCEP ATP-III an explicit demonstration of insulin resistance is not required.

In contrast, the WHO guidelines view insulin resistance as a required component for diagnosis. In addition to insulin resistance, two other risk factors are required for the diagnosis of the metabolic syndrome. Microalbumineria has also been added to the list as a criterion.

The AACE criteria seem to be a reconciliation between the NCEP ATP-III and the WHO guidelines. Although the clinical criteria are listed, the number of risk factors required to claim the existence of metabolic syndrome are not specified and left to clinical judgment. Both AACE and WHO guidelines included insulin resistance measurement methods which are beyond routine clinical assessment. Indeed, for these two authorities, values derived from an oral glucose tolerance test are among the risk factors for the metabolic syndrome. Although these measurements give additional information, they add time and cost to clinical practice. Therefore, the NCEP ATP-III guidelines may be more suitable on a clinical basis.

Table 1. National Cholesterol Education Program's Adult Treatment Panel-III report (NCEP ATP-III) clinical criteria for the metabolic syndrome (NCEP, 2002).

Risk Factors	Defining Level
Abdominal obesity, given as waist circumference	
Men	>102 cm (>40 in)
Women	>88 cm (>35 in)
Triglycerides	≥150 mg/dL (≥1.7 mmol/L)
HDL cholesterol	
Men	<40 mg/dL (<1.0 mmol/L)
Women	<50 mg/dL (<1.3 mmol/L)
Blood pressure	≥130/≥85 mm Hg
Fasting glucose	≥110 mg/dL (≥ 6.1 mmol/L)

2.2. Myocardial Aging

Unlike systolic ventricular function, which is relatively well preserved with aging, diastolic function declines after the age of 30 years (Benjamin et al, 1992). Even in the absence of cardiovascular disease, the incidence of diastolic heart failure increases exponentially with age (Grossman et al, 1991).

It is unclear whether the age-associated decline in diastolic function is caused by aging itself or by other factors which are associated with age. Many of these factors are now being considered risk factors for cardiovascular diseases, such as insulin resistance, metabolic syndrome and degree of cardiovascular fitness. All these variables are known to be associated with diastolic function.

The main functional change of age-related diastolic dysfunction is an increase in myocardial stiffness resulting from modifications in ventricular passive diastolic properties (Bhatia et al, 2006).

Table 2. World Health Organization (WHO) clinical criteria for the metabolic syndrome (WHO, 1998).

Insulin resistance, identified by 1 of the following:

- Type 2 diabetes
- Impaired fasting glucose
- Impaired glucose tolerance
- Or for those with normal fasting glucose levels (<110 mg/dL), glucose uptake below the lowest quartile for background population under investigation under hyperinsulinemic, euglycemic conditions

Plus any 2 of the following:

- Antihypertensive medication and/or high blood pressure (≥14C mm Hg systolic or ≥90 mm Hg diastolic)
- Plasma triglycerides ≥150 mg/dL (≥1.7 mmol/L)
- HDL cholesterol <35 mg/dL (<0.9 mmol/L) in men or <39 mg/dL (1.0 mmol/L) in women
- BMI >30 kg/m^2 and/or waist:hip ratio >0.9 in men, >0.85 in women
- Urinary albumin excretion rate ≥20 µg/min or albumin:creatine ratio ≥30 mg/g

Table 3. American Association of Clinical Endocrinologists (AACE) clinical criteria for the metabolic syndrome (AACE, 2003).

Risk Factor Components	Cutpoints for abnormality
Overweight/obesity	BMI ≥ 25 kg/m^2
Elevated triglycerides	≥150 mg/dL (1.7 mmol/L)
Low HDL choleterol	
Men	<40 mg/dL (1.0 mmol/L)
Women	<50 mg/dL (1.3 mmol/L)
Elevated blood pressure	≥130/85 mm Hg
2-Hour postglucose challenge	>140 mg/dL
Fasting glucose	Between 110 and 126 mg/dL
Other risk factors	Family history of type 2 diabetes, hypertension, or CVD, polycystic ovary syndrome, sedentary lifestyle, advancing age, ethnic groups having high risk for type 2 diabetes or CVD

Diastolic heart failure (DHF) is characterized by a nondilated left ventricle and/or a concentric left ventricle hypertrophy or remodeling, and it is principally caused by left ventricular diastolic dysfunction, where left ventricular function is in the normal range, while abnormalities in left ventricular diastolic properties (delayed active relaxation and elevated passive stiffness) predominate and determine increased end-diastolic pressure (Maeder, et al. 2009).

The pathology hallmark is an increase in fibrillar collagen, which is a component of the extracellular matrix (ECM), which is postulated to be a determinant of myocardial stiffness. Furthermore, some have suggested that collagen cross-linkings, rather than total collagen or types of collagen, are even more important at determining chamber stiffness in the heart (Zile et al, 2005).

There are also important mechanisms intrinsically related to cardiomyocytes. The main intrinsic myocyte factors include abnormalities in the sarcolemmal calcium channels, the sarcoplasmic reticulum calcium ATPase, and also in the phosphorylation of some important proteins. These alterations lead to an increased cytosolic calcium concentration during early and late diastole; thus, the remaining higher cytosolic calcium concentration could impair the ability of cardiac myocyte to relax and lengthen throughout the entire diastole (Zile et al, 2005).

2.3. Diastolic Heart Failure

Diastole is the period of time during which the myocardium loses its ability to generate force and shorten and returns to an unstressed length and force (Zile et al, 2002). Diastolic dysfunction appears when this process is prolonged, slowed, or incomplete.

It is traditionally divided into four phases, i.e. isovolumetric relaxation, early diastolic filling, diastasis and atrial contraction. Many factors determine LV filling, like myocardial relaxation, atrial contraction, diastolic restoring forces, pericardial restraint, myocardial irrigation, cardiac conduction system and others. These factors overlap in time and are influenced by each other, by LV systolic function, heart rate, and by the cardiac conduction system (Gilbert, 1989). Their final combined effect is on the transmitral pressure gradient, which actually determines LV filling.

In the clinical definition most often used, diastole is delineated by the time interval between closure of the aortic valve and closure of the mitral valve.

Diastolic dysfunction refers to a condition in which abnormalities in mechanical function are present during diastole.

The causes of diastolic dysfunction may be subdivided into a decrease in passive myocardial diastolic compliance, and impairment in active LV relaxation.

Abnormalities in diastolic function may occur in the presence or absence of a clinical syndrome of heart failure and with normal or abnormal systolic function. Therefore, whereas diastolic dysfunction describes an abnormal mechanical property, diastolic heart failure describes a clinical syndrome.

Diastolic heart failure is increasingly recognized as an important clinical syndrome, but the criteria for diagnosis are subject to debate.

Practical recommendations for diagnosis have been made by both the Canadian Cardiovascular Society and the American College of Cardiology in a joint effort with the American Heart Association. According to these groups, a diagnosis of diastolic heart failure should be considered when there are signs and symptoms of heart failure (e.g., fatigue, pulmonary congestion and dependent edema) and when there is objective evidence of a normal or near normal ejection fraction, either with or without demonstrated diastolic abnormalities, and without valvular defects. Patients should also be free of pericardial disease or a systemic condition (e.g., anemia or renal failure) that could explain their heart failure (Cosson et al, 2003). This is the definition of diastolic heart failure that we have adopted for our review.

3. Metabolic Syndrome, Myocardial Aging, and Diastolic Dysfunction

3.1. Metabolic Syndrome and Aging

Based on the NCEP ATP-III definition, the prevalence of the metabolic syndrome has been established in the Third National Health and Nutrition Examination Survey (NHANES III). Overall, the unadjusted prevalence of the metabolic syndrome was approximately 22% in this US adult population. However, the prevalence of this condition increases with age both in men and women to reach almost 45% for subjects aged above 60 years (Figure 1). Considering the epidemic of obesity, these numbers are very likely to be higher today compared to the estimates derived from 1988-1994 NHANES III survey.

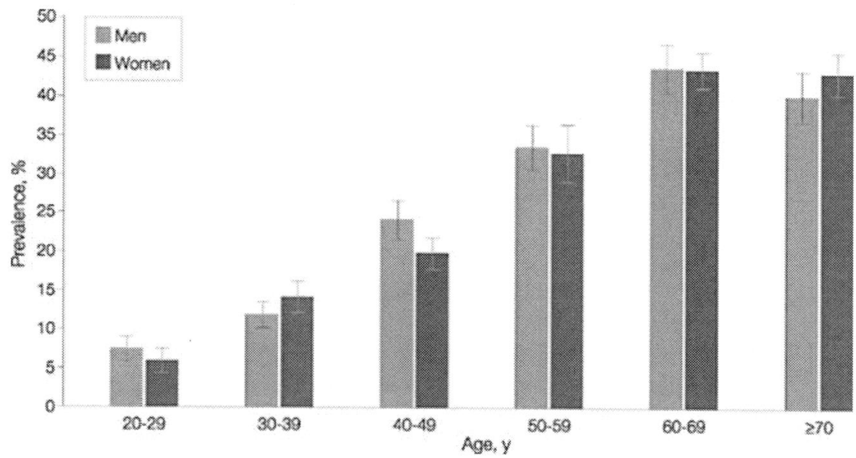

Adapted from Ford et al, 2002.

Figure 1. Age-specific prevalence of the metabolic syndrome among 8814 US adults aged at least 20 years, by sex, National Health and Nutrition Examination Survey III, 1988-1994.

It has been recognized that Insulin Resistance has a central role in regulating biological aging, by increasing the formation of Reactive Oxygen Species (ROS) and Advance Glucose Endproducts (AGEs), key points for each of the two main theories of aging: oxidative stress and protein glycation, respectively.

3.2. Metabolic Syndrome and Diastolic Left Ventricular Dysfunction

Left ventricular (LV) remodeling in type 2 diabetes, includes increased LV mass, wall thicknesses, arterial stiffness, reduced LV systolic chamber and myocardial function (Devereux el al, 2000). LV mass and wall thickness increase with worsening glucose intolerance (Rutter et al, 2003). Diabetes mellitus, especially with lower glycaemic control, is independently associated with abnormal LV relaxation, similar to the impaired relaxation associated with hypertension (Liu et al, 2001).

DM2 is independently associated with a 2.0 times greater risk of LV systolic dysfunction and a 2.4 times greater risk of LV diastolic dysfunction. This may explain the increased risk of systolic and diastolic heart failure in elderly individuals with DM2 (Henry, et al, 2008).

Blood pressure (BP) overload explains only in part the changes in LV structure in subjects with hypertension, because the proportion of LV mass variability accounted for in these subjects by BP, either clinically or ambulatory, is small (Devereux et al, 1995). Insulin could be involved in the pathogenesis of essential hypertension (Denker et al,1992).

Diabetic patients can develop heart failure related to vascular pathology mainly associated with hypertension and coronary artery disease, but these patients can also develop a condition named diabetic cardiomyopathy. This is type of cardiomyopathy, diagnosed when ventricular dysfunction develops in patients with diabetes in the absence of coronary atherosclerosis and hypertension. It refers to a disease process which affects the myocardium in diabetic patients causing a wide range of structural abnormalities eventually leading to left ventricular hypertrophy and diastolic and systolic dysfunction or a combination of these (Poornima, et al., 2006).

A significant number of diabetic patients exhibit diabetic cardiomyopathy. Accumulating data from experimental, pathological, epidemiological, and clinical studies have shown that diabetes mellitus results in cardiac functional and structural changes, independent of hypertension, coronary artery disease, or any other known cardiac disease, which support the existence of diabetic cardiomyopathy (Fang, et al., 2004).

Verdecchia et al demonstrated, in 1999, that insulin and IGF-1 are important determinants of LV mass and geometry in subjects with essential hypertension and normal glucose tolerance, and that this relation is independent of sex, weight, and office or ambulatory BP.

Insulin and IGF-1 could lead to increased LV mass through different basic effects on left ventricular geometry. An inverse association has been noted between insulin sensitivity, measured by the glucose clamp technique, and LV wall thickness in subjects with essential hypertension (Lind et al, 1995).

The formation of Reactive Oxygen Species (ROS) and Advance Glucose Endproducts (AGEs), cited above, both related to aging and metabolic syndrome, causes microangiopathy, increased extracellular collagen deposition and abnormalities in calcium transport, abnormalities that culminate in ventricular diastolic dysfunction.

Other mechanism that may contribute to myocardial dysfunctions (especially diastolic ones) in dysmetabolic disorders, including type 2 diabetes mellitus, obesity, and the metabolic syndrome is the intracellular deposition of lipids in the myocites. Plasma triglycerides levels show a strong relationship with impaired left ventricular relaxation in human beings. Mechanisms whereby intracellular lipid accumulation may alter left ventricular diastolic function include one or more of the following:

(1) a relative state of energy depletion resulting from the favored oxidation of a less efficient fuel (ie, fatty acids) that compromises diastolic relaxation, an energy-dependent process;
(2) increased intracellular lipid deposition leading to structural changes favoring left ventricular hypertrophy, thus, resulting in secondary diastolic dysfunction;
(3) accumulation of toxic lipid intermediaries and / or generation of reactive oxygen species leading to myocellular dysfunction and/or apoptosis; or
(4) intracellular lipids disrupt excitation / contraction coupling by effects on ion channels.

Further studies are needed to address the precise molecular mechanisms mediating the association between plasma TG levels and diastolic function (de las Fuentes, et al, 2005).

4. Cardiac Rehabilitation in Insulin Resistance-Related Diastolic Heart Failure

Patients with heart failure have an inadequate increase in cardiac output during exercise. Diastolic Heart Failure is associated with significant physical activity intolerance, involving intrinsic and extrinsic components of left ventricular myocytes, which determines decreased left ventricular diastolic compliance, decreased aortic distensibility, and increased systolic arterial pressure during exercise, cardiac dyssynchrony and possibly an alteration in the skeletal muscle metabolism and activity. In fact, when DHF patients are put in exercise, they may not be able to increase cardiac output without a markedly increase in the diastolic pressures because of an impaired left ventricular relaxation, as well as a reduction in end-diastolic volume due to a shortened diastole during tachycardia (Piña, et al., 2003).

However when exercise training is safe it provides several benefits to these patients. Exercise training improves left ventricular function and hemodynamic status, including endothelial functioning and vasodilatation, skeletal muscle metabolism, autonomic nervous system modulation of the cardiovascular function, and even the plasmatic levels of several inflammatory mediators like necrosis factor-α, interleukin-6 and nitric oxide, which may lead to better functional capacity (Wielenga, et al., 1997; Piña, et al., 2003).

4.1. Evaluating Metabolic Syndrome

Managing the metabolic syndrome components in an integrated approach may contribute to cardiac rehabilitation in patients with diastolic heart failure in many ways. The control of its components may improve diastolic relaxation through several mechanisms. All of them can be reached by pharmacologic or non–pharmacologic interventions. Exercise training will be explored separately.

Obesity and overweight: Losing weight by itself can ameliorate diastolic heart failure by both direct and indirect mechanisms. First, weight reduction would decrease the need for a continuously elevated cardiac output at rest which would improve symptoms in heart failure. Second, this approach also contributes to better control of all of the metabolic syndrome components.

A Hypertension: Tight control of blood pressure would prevent myocardial remodeling and even regress, to some degree, this process, improving diastolic function.

B Insulin resistance and diabetes: Glycemic control has the potential to decelerate myocardial aging and, additionally, improve diastolic function both by regressing cardiac microangiopathy and intracellular glucose utilization by the myocardial cell.

C Hypertrigliceridemia: Controlling triglyceride levels may improve the diastolic function, as seen above. Plasma triglycerides levels show a strong relationship with impaired left ventricular relaxation

4.2. Exercise Training

Exercise is an essential part in the cardiac rehabilitation plan of the patient with diastolic heart failure that is insulin-resistance associated. Independent of weight reduction, dynamic exercise is able to improve insulin resistance, diastolic function, and peripheral energy utilization, all mechanisms collaborating in the rehabilitation on diastolic heart failure.

4.2.1. Effects of Exercise Upon the aged Myocardium

Studies suggest that bed rest deconditioning impairs endurance while training improves cardiac compliance (Levine, et al, 1991, 1997).

A sedentary lifestyle is associated with a decline of ventricular compliance, leading to higher cardiac filling pressures and lower stroke volumes for a given filling volume compared with age-matched athletes or young individuals. Prolonged, sustained endurance training preserves ventricular compliance with aging and may be an important approach to reduce the probability of heart failure with aging (Arbab-Zadeh et al, 2004).

Brenner et al, in 2001, found that 12 weeks of exercise training in the aged rats largely reversed the age-associated impairment in early diastolic filling. The underlying molecular mechanism for this improvement could be either reversal of the age associated changes that resulted in the impaired diastolic function, or alternatively, some beneficial effect of training on diastolic function in general.

In isometrically contracting papillary muscle and trabeculae carneae from rats, age-associated slowing of contraction and relaxation can be reversed with exercise training (Spurgeon, et al, 1983).

Takemoto et al, in 1992, reported that trained subjects had better resting diastolic function than age- matched untrained subjects. In a longitudinal study, Levy et al, in 1993, reported that training improved early diastolic filling in older men as assessed with radionuclide ventriculography. Even in the presence of dilated cardiomyopathy, exercise training demonstrated improvement in resting BP (Belardinelli, et al, 1995).

4.2.2. Exercise training and the components of the metabolic syndrome

A. Obesity

The characteristic feature of obesity associated with the metabolic syndrome is the android or abdominal obesity type. Both genetic and environmental factors contribute to the development of obesity and the distribution of body fat.

Treatment of obesity is simple in theory, but not in practice. This statement is nicely supported by the vast amount of published studies evaluating various treatment modalities – and the worldwide increase in the prevalence of obesity.

Exercise preserves lean body mass, unlike dieting alone. This is crucial since the major determinant of the 24h energy expendure (EE) is the fat-free body mass, accounting for about 80% of the variance observed in 24hEE between individuals (Horton et al, 1985).

There are some differences between types of exercise performed. A combination of resistance training and aerobic endurance exercise appears to be most efficient in preserving fat-free body mass, compared to aerobic endurance exercise alone. Thus, an exercise program for the treatment of obesity should include both aerobic endurance training and resistance training (American College of Sports Medicine, 1990)

B. Hypertension

Epidemiological and clinical studies indicate a lower incidence of hypertension in physically active individuals, in all age groups. Likewise positive effects of physical activity and exercise on blood pressure have been reported. Exercise has shown to prevent age-associated increases in blood pressure (Blair et al, 1984)

A meta-analysis of 25 longitudinal studies examining the antihypertensive effects of exercise, showed reductions in resting systolic and diastolic blood pressure of 11 and 8 mmHg, respectively. In 67% of the experimental groups statistically significant reductions were noted in systolic blood pressure; the corresponding value for the diastolic blood pressure was 70% (Hagberg et al, 1990).

The overall impression from the published studies is that regular exercise training provides a modest antihypertensive effect and the use of exercise therapy for the treatment of hypertension is most beneficial in the early stages of hypertension as well as for the prevention of hypertension.

C. Insulin resistance and glucose intolerance

The association of physical inactivity and insulin resistance was first suggested over 60 years ago (Blotner et al, 1945)

Since then, both cross-sectional and intervention studies have addressed the association between physical activity and insulin sensitivity. In cross-sectional studies, endurance athletes demonstrate lower serum insulin levels in the fasting and postprandial state, and greater insulin sensitivity compared to their sedentary counterparts. Master athletes also seem to be protected against a deterioration of glucose tolerance normally associated with aging (Rogers et al, 1990). To what extent greater insulin sensitivity in the athletes is due to natural selection and reflects genetic endowment rather than the effect of physical training cannot be firmly established from cross-sectional studies. In intervention studies the effects of both acute and chronic exercise on insulin sensitivity have been assessed.

It has been estimated that at least 25% of the incidence of NIDDM may be attributable to a sedentary lifestyle. Consequently the beneficial effects of exercise and physical activity in the prevention of NIDDM are numerous.

If exercise training is discontinued, the improvements gained in both insulin sensitivity and glucose tolerance will vanish within a few days. Improved insulin sensitivity has been demonstrated 12–48 h after the exercise bout, but is virtually unmeasurable 3– 5 days after the last exercise session (Mikinis et al, 1988). However, this can be rapidly regained by one single bout of exercises. If physical exercise is minimal during leisure time, insulin sensitivity is low, and a few days bed rest is associated with substantial insulin resistance.

Insulin resistance is often present in individuals who are not overtly obese, such as first-degree relatives of NIDDM subjects. These 'metabolically obese normal-weight' individuals appear to be quite common in the general population, and they could be an important target population for exercise therapy, for the prevention of the metabolic syndrome. Also, the potential role of a diminished physical work capacity in the pathogenesis of insulin resistance among first-degree relatives of NIDDM subjects has been stressed (Nyholm et al,1996).

D. Dyslipidaemia

Dyslipidaemia associated with the metabolic syndrome is primarily characterized by hypertriglyceridemia and low levels of HDL-cholesterol.

The effects of exercise on lipid and lipoprotein profiles are fairly well known. Early studies emphasizing the differences in total cholesterol and triglycerides between individuals involved in endurance type exercise and sedentary subjects, have been confirmed by later studies. According to the present consensus, physically active individuals have higher levels of HDL- and HDL2-cholesterol and lower levels of triglycerides, VLDL- and dense LDL-cholesterol, compared to sedentary individuals. Furthermore, intervention studies have shown that unfavorable lipid and lipoprotein profiles respond favorably to exercise training (Durstine et al, 1994)

It is likely that subjects with the metabolic syndrome would also benefit from exercise as do other individuals with dyslipidaemia. Exercise training increases the ability of muscle tissue to take up and oxidize non-esterified fatty acids and increases the activity of lipoprotein lipase (LPL) in muscle. The combined effects of exercise and diet among NIDDM subjects resulted in a decrease in total and LDL-cholesterol, while HDL-cholesterol increased. However, it is difficult to separate dietary influences from the effects of exercise on serum lipids and lipoproteins. Both the separate and combined effects of diet and exercise in reducing body weight and improving serum lipid and lipoprotein profiles among overweight subjects have been evaluated. Both treatment modalities caused significant increases in HDL1-, HDL2- and HDL3-cholesterol and decreases in triglyceride levels (Eriksson et al, 1997). Aerobic endurance exercise training and a low fat diet can normalize the metabolic profile of obese women, even if their adiposity remains higher than that of lean women. In the studies by Lampman and Schteingart (1991) exercise training alone increased insulin sensitivity, improved glucose tolerance, and lowered triglyceride and cholesterol levels among non-diabetic, non-obese subjects with hypertriglyceridaemia. However, these improvements did not occur when exercise training alone was performed by similar patients with impaired glucose tolerance.

Considering the evidence indicated above, it is very likely that exercise, either alone or combined with proper diet, is effective in improving serum lipid and lipoprotein profiles among subjects with the metabolic syndrome. However, it is difficult to distinguish the independent effect of exercise on serum lipids and lipoprotein profile from the effects of other beneficial health habits associated with regular exercise. Obesity, smoking, and excessive use of dietary fat are less prevalent among physically active subjects.

5. Conclusion

Several lines of evidences indicate that metabolic syndrome accelerate myocardial aging, increasing the risk of age-related diastolic dysfunction and consequent heart failure. Adequate management of the metabolic syndrome and its components, including both pharmacological and non-pharmacological interventions, such as aerobic exercise, may have important implications not only in preventing age-related diastolic dysfunction, but also in cardiac rehabilitation.

6. References

[1] American Association of Clinical Endocrinologists (AACE) consensus conference on the insulin resistance syndrome: 25-26 August 2002, Washington, DC. *Diabetes Care.*, 2003, 26(4), 1297-303.

[2] American College of Sports Medicine. The recommended quantity and quality of exercise for developing and maintaining cardiorespiratory and muscular fitness in healthy adults. *Med Sci Sports Exerc*, 1990, 22, 265-274.

[3] Arbab-Zadeh, et al. Aging and Left Ventricular Compliance. *Circulation.*, 2004, 110, 1799-1805.

[4] Belardinelli, R; Georgiou, D; Cianci, G; et al. Exercise training improves left ventricular diastolic filling in patients with dilated cardiomyopathy: clinical and prognostic implications. *Circulation.*, 1995, 91, 2775-2784.

[5] Benjamin, EJ; Levy, D; Anderson, KM; et al. Determinants of Doppler indexes of left ventricular diastolic function in normal subjects (the Framingham Heart Study). *Am J Cardiol.*, 1992, 70, 508-515.

[6] Blair SN; Goodyear, NN; Gibbons, W; Cooper, KH. Physical fitness and incidence of hypertension in healthy normotensive men and women. *JAMA*, 1984, 252, 487-490.

[7] Blotner, H. Effects of prolonged physical inactivation tolerance of sugar. *Arch Int Med*, 1945, 75, 39-44.

[8] Brenner, et al. Exercise Training Attenuates Age-Associated Diastolic Dysfunction in Rats. *Circulation*, 2001, 104, 221-226.

[9] Cosson, S; Kevorkian, JP. Left ventricular diastolic dysfunction: an early sign of diabetic cardiomyopathy? *Diabetes Metab*, 2003, 29,455-66.

[10] Denker, PS; Pollock, VE. Fasting serum insulin levels in essential hypertension: a meta-analysis. *Arch Intern Med.*, 1992, 152, 1649-1651.

[11] Devereux, RB; Roman, MJ; Paranicas, M; et al. Impact of diabetes on cardiac structure and function: the Strong Heart Study. *Circulation*, 2000, 101, 2271-6.

[12] Devereux, RB; Roman, MJ. Hypertensive cardiac hypertrophy: pathophysiologic and clinical characteristics. In: Laragh JH; Brenner BM; eds. Hypertension: Pathophysiology, Diagnosis, Treatment (2nd ed), Raven Press, Cary, NC (1995), 409-432.

[13] Durstine, JL; Haskell, WL. Effects of exercise on plasma lipids and lipoproteins. *Exerc Sport Sci Rev*, 1994, 22, 477-521.

[14] Eriksson, J; Taimela, S; Koivisto, VA. Exercise and the metabolic syndrome. *Diabetologia*, 1997, 40, 125-35.

[15] Fang, ZY; Prins, JB; Marwick, TH. Diabetic Cardiomyopathy: Evidence, Mechanisms, and Therapeutic Implications. *Endocrine Reviews*, 2004, 25(4), 543-567.

[16] Ford, ES; Giles, WH; Dietz, WH; et al. Prevalence of the Metabolic Syndrome Among US Adults. Findings From the Third National Health and Nutrition Examination Survey. *JAMA*, 2002, 287, 356-359.

[17] Gilbert, JC; Glantz, SA. Determinants of LV filling and of the diastolic pressure-volume relation. *Circ Res*, 1989, 64, 827-52.

[18] Grossman W. Diastolic dysfunction in congestive heart failure. *N Engl J Med.*, 1991, 325, 1557-1564.

[19] Hagberg, JM. Exercise; fitness and hypertension. In: Bouchard C (ed) Exercise, fitness and health: a consensus of current knowledge. *Human Kinetic Books*, 1990, Champaign, Illinois.

[20] Henry, RM; Paulus, WJ; Kamp, O; et al. Deteriorating glucose tolerance status is associated with left ventricular dysfunction--the Hoorn Study. *Neth J Med.*, 2008, Mar; 66(3), 110-7.

[21] Horton, ES; et al. Metabolic aspects of exercise andweight reduction. *Med Sci Sports Exerc.*, 1985, 18, 10-18.

[22] Hypertension: Pathophysiology, Diagnosis and Management. 2nd ed.New York, NY: Raven Press, Ltd; 1995, 409-424.

[23] Lampman, RM; Schteingart, DE. Effects of exercise training on glucose control, lipid metabolism, and insulin sensitivity in hypertriglyceridemia and non-insulin dependent diabetes mellitus. Med Sci Sports Exerc 1991, 23, 703-712.

[24] Levine, BD; Lane, LD; Buckey, JC; et al. Left ventricular pressure-volume and Frank-Starling relations in endurance athletes: implications for orthostatic tolerance and exercise performance. *Circulation.*, 1991, 84, 1016-1023.

[25] Levine, BD; Zuckerman, JH; Pawelczyk, JA. Cardiac atrophy after bed-rest deconditioning: a nonneural mechanism for orthostatic intolerance. *Circulation.*, 1997, 96, 517-525.

[26] Levy, WC; Cerqueira, MD; Abrass, IB; et al. Endurance exercise training augments diastolic filling at rest and during exercise in healthy young and older men. *Circulation.*, 1993, 88, 116-126.

[27] Lind, L; Andersson, PE; Andre´n, B; Hanni, A; Lithell, HO. Left ventricular hypertrophy in hypertension is associated with the insulin resistance metabolic syndrome. *J Hypertens.*, 1995, 13, 433-43.

[28] de las Fuentes, L; Waggoner, A; Brown, A; et al. Plasma Triglyceride Level is an Independent Predictor of Altered Left Ventricular Relaxation. *J Am Soc Echocardiogr*, 2005, 18, 1285-1291.

[29] Liu, JE; Palmieri, V; Roman, MJ; et al. The impact of diabetes on left ventricular filling pattern in normotensive and hypertensive adults: the Strong Heart Study. *J Am Coll Cardiol*, 2001, 37, 1943-9.

[30] Maeder, MT; Kaye, DM. Heart failure with normal left ventricular ejection fraction. J. Am. Coll. Cardiol. 2009; 51(11): 905-918.

[31] Mikinis, KJ; Sonne, B; Farrell, PA; Tronier, B; Galbo, H. Effect of physical exercise on sensitivity and responsiveness to insulin in humans. *Am J Physiol*, 1988, 254, E248–E259.

[32] National Cholesterol Education Program (NCEP) Expert Panel on Detection, Evaluation, and Treatment of High Blood Cholesterol in Adults (Adult Treatment Panel III – ATP III). Third Report of the National Cholesterol Education Program (NCEP) Panel on Detection, Evaluation, and Treatment of High Blood Cholesterol in Adults (Adult

Treatment Panel III) final report. Circulation., 2002, 17, 106(25):3143-421.

[33] Nyholm, B; Mengel, A; Nielsen, S; et al. Insulin resistance in relatives of NIDDM patients: the role of physical fitness and muscle metabolism. Diabetologia, 1996, 39, 813-822.

[34] Paolo Verdecchia, Gianpaolo Reboldi, Giuseppe Schillaci, Claudia Borgioni Antonella Ciucci, Maria Pia Telera, Fausto Santeusanio, Carlo Porcellati and Paolo Brunetti. Circulating Insulin and Insulin Growth Factor-1 Are Independent Determinants of Left Ventricular Mass and Geometry in Essential Hypertension. *Circulation*, 1999, 100, 1802-1807.

[35] Piña, IL; Chair Writing Group Apstein, CS; Balady, GJ; Belardinelli, R; Chaitman, BR; Duscha, BD; Fletcher, BJ; Fleg, JL; Myers, JN; Sullivan, MJ. Exercise and heart failure: a statement from the American Heart Association Committee on Exercise, Rehabilitation, and Prevention. *Circulation*, 2003, 107(8), 1210-1225.

[36] Poornima, IG; Parikh, P; Shannon, RP. Diabetic Cardiomyopathy - The Search for a Unifying Hypothesis. *Circulation Research.*, 2006; 98;596-605.

[37] Rogers, MA; King, DS; Hagberg, JM; Ehsani, AA; Holloszy, JO. Effect of 10 days of physical inactivity on glucose tolerance in master athletes. J Appl Physiol. 1990, 68(5), 1833-7.

[38] Rutter, MK; Parise, H; Benjamin, EJ; et al. Impact of glucose intolerance and insulin resistance on cardiac structure and function: sexrelated differences in the Framingham Heart Study. *Circulation*, 2003, 107, 448–54.

[39] Spurgeon, HA; Steinbach, MF; Lakatta, EG. Chronic exercise prevents characteristic age-related changes in rat cardiac contraction. *Am J Physiol.*, 1983, 244, H513-H518.

[40] Takemoto, KA; Bernstein, L; Lopez, JF; et al. Abnormalities of diastolic filling of the left ventricle associated with aging are less pronounced inexercise-trained individuals. *Am Heart J.*, 1992, 124, 143-148.

[41] Wielenga, RP; Coats, AJS; Mosterd, WL; Huisveld IA. The role of exercise training in chronic heart failure. *Heart*, 1997, 78(5), 431-436.

[42] World Health Organization (WHO). Definition, diagnosis and classification of diabetes mellitus and its complications. Part 1:

diagnosis and classification of diabetes mellitus provisional report of a WHO consultation. *Diabet Med*, 15, 539-553, 1998.

[43] Zile, MR; Brutsaert, DL. New concepts in diastolic dysfunction and diastolic heart failure: Part I: diagnosis, prognosis, and measurements of diastolic function. *Circulation*, 2002, 19, 1387-93.

In: Cardiac Rehabilitaiton
Editor: J. T. Halliday, pp. 165-184
ISBN: 978-1-60741-918-1

Chapter VII

Asymptomatic Upper-Extremity Deep Vein Thrombosis Catheter-Related and Pulmonary Embolism after Cardiac Surgery . A Prospective Study of 1000 Patients Admitted to Intensive Cardiac Rehabilitation

Rino Frizzelli**, Ornella Tortelli, Cleante Scarduelli , Redenta Ghirardi, Claudio Pinzi, Emanuele Bassi

Division of Cardiorespiratory Physiopathology and Rehabilitation Unit, Multifunctional Rehabilitation Hospital, Bozzolo, Mantova, (Italy)

* Correspondence Rino Frizzelli,MD, Director of Cardiopulmonary Rehabilitation, Presidio Ospedaliero di Bozzolo, via XXV aprile 71, 46012 Bozzolo (Mantova), Italy, Phone 0036-0376.909240- (Phone home 0036-0375 88844) fax 0036-0376 909208, e-mail: rino.frizzelli@aopoma.it

Abstract

Introduction

Venous thromboembolism (VTE) is an important cause of morbidity and mortality after many general surgical procedures and can be a complication of central venous catheterization(CVC) .

In cardiac surgery the CVC is frequently placed in the right internal jugular vein, but procedure has still not been properly assessed as regards either the risk of deep vein thrombosis catheter- related (DVT–CVC related) and Pulmonary embolism (PE).We assessed the impact of right internal jugular vein CVC-related DVT and the risk of PE in patients after coronary artery bypass grafts (CABG), valve replacement surgery, or both; we also assessed therapeutic options.

Material and Methods

We considered 1000 patients after cardiac surgery and admitted to intensive cardiac rehabilitation 5 to 7 days later (mean 5.8);960 were enrolled.

All had CVC in right internal jugular vein: a triple-lumen central venous catheter 14 gauge was inserted immediately before surgery and removed 3 to 4 days later;within 3 days after admission the patients were checked by ultrasonography (US) exploring neck vessels.

DVT diagnosed was classified as at low risk of embolism when it was only a small strip less than 2 cm long (limited) or at high risk of embolism when it was free-floating or sub-occlusive the lumen. PE had been confirmed by pulmonary angio-CT scan.

Results

461 patients (48%) had asymptomatic CVC-related DVT. None of the patients with CVC-related DVT and anticoagulant therapy presented clinical signs or symptoms of PE while in rehabilitation, or after three months. Among the patients with CVC-related DVT receiving antiplatelet and considered at low risk ,PE was seen in the six cases; among all those considered at high risk of embolism , the antiplatelet was replaced with low-molecular-weight fractionated heparin and warfarin (INR 2,5-3,5), continued for at least three months or until there were no

longer any US signs of thrombosis. This group had no cases of clinically manifest PE either while in hospital or at three months.

Discussion

Very little is known about the prevalence of thrombotic events in CVC-related DVT of the neck after cardiac surgery. In the present study with several types of heart surgery, 48% had DVT related to a CVC in the right internal jugular vein; this is significantly higher than the figure for lower-extremity DVT in the same type of population . About 1,200,000 heart operations are performed every year in the U.S.A.; therefore, we can assume that more than 500,000 heart operations each year may be complicated with CVC-related DVT.

The causes or factors responsible for this complication are still not clear, just as the real reason why the thrombus forms is not known. Controversy also surrounds the question of how best to prevent CVC-related DVT:the utility for preventing CVC-related DVT with unfractionated heparin and warfarin remains to be established .Our findings suggest that neither heparin given during surgery nor anticoagulant therapy with heparin and warfarin immediately after surgery are very reliable for preventing venous thrombosis; early antiplatelet therapy also had no significant preventive effect. Anticoagulation with warfarin does seem to prevent clinically manifest PE in all patients with CVC-related DVT, regardless of type of thrombus or heart surgery. In addition, sonographic screening of the CVC removal in intensive cardiac unit may be useful for avoiding PE after CVC-related DVT.

Introduction

Central venous catheterization (CVC) is becoming increasingly in a wide variety of patients for indications such a monitoring of hemodynamic variables, administration of drugs, hemoderivatives, total parenteral nutrition and hemodialysis [1].

Unfortunately, the advantages secured by the extensive use of CVC are associated with adverse events that are hazardouse to patients and expensive to treat [2-3]. More than 15 percent of patients who receive these catheters have complications: mechanical complications are reported to occur in 5 to 19 percent of patients and infections complications in 5 to 26 percent;

furthermore,patients who require CVC can be at high risk for catheter-related thrombosis and thrombotic complications in 2 to 26 percent [4-7], but it varies according to the side of insertion .

The complications rates affects a significant number of patients because an estimated more than five million CVCs are performed every year in the United States [8].

In cardiac surgery, the CVC is normally placed in the right internal jugular vein, and left there for 3 or 4 days, but the procedure has still not been completely evaluated with regard to either the risk of deep venous thrombosis (DVT), i.e. CVC-related DVT, or secondary pulmonary embolism (PE). Most reports describe only lower-extremity DVT after coronary artery bypass surgery [9-11], and upper extremity thrombi are usually found in the axillary, subclavian or brachiocephalic veins[12-13], not in the right internal jugular vein .

The clinical importance of catheter-related thrombosis remains undefined, although all thromboses have the potential to embolize[14]: this study assessed the impact of right internal jugular vein CVC-related DVT and the risk of PE in patients after coronary artery bypass grafts (CABG), valve replacement surgery, or both. We also assessed therapeutic options.

Materials and Methods

Setting: Intensive Cardiac Rehabilitation Unit

Patient selection

We considered 1000 consecutive patients discharged after heart surgery and admitted to intensive cardiac rehabilitation 5–7 days (mean 5.8). A total of 40 had to be excluded because they had a CVC in place for more than a week, thrombogenic diathesis or haemostatic disorders (prior history of DVT, embolism, thrombocytosis [600,000 mmc-1] or malignancies(Figure1).

This left 960 (675 male, 285 female, mean 67.7 ± 10.2 years); 624 had bypass surgery, 268 valve surgery, and 68 the combination (Tab.I).

All had a CVC in the right internal jugular vein: a triple lumen central venous catheter 14 gauge was inserted immediately before surgery and removed 3–4 days later (Figure2).

Perioperative prophylaxis for DVT was comparable and homogeneous in various centers. After removal of chest tubes, the patients received subcutaeous calcium heparin at a dose of 200 IU/kg daily for at least 48–72 h after surgery, adjusted to maintain the activated partial thromboplastin time in the range of 1.5–2.5 times the control range. Warfarin was tapered in and continued as maintenance therapy (defined by an international normalized ratio >2) in cardiac prosthetic valve or CABG with atrial fibrillation; calcium heparin was replaced with an antiplatelet agent (aspirin 100 mg daily) in CABG with sinus rhythm [15-16].

Upon admission to intensive cardiac rehabilitation, none of these patients was known to have a CVC-related DVT.All participating patients gave a written informed consent and were studied according to a protocol approved by the Institutional Ethics Committee.

Within 3 days after admission, a single operator studied all patients by ultrasonography (US) using a convex Esaote 7.5 MHz sound with color Doppler, with the patient supine, exploring neck vessels and displaying the cross and longitudinal sections of the right jugular-brachiocephalic venous area. The examination was interpreted separately by two independent observers who were cardiologists. The diagnosis of DVT was made only when both observers were in complete agreement. A clinical evaluation and US examination were scheduled at 3 months. All patients were available for follow-up.

Criteria for CVC-Related DVT

At the US examination, all patients still had slough signs on the skin over the right jugular where the catheter had been inserted. A DVT was diagnosed based on simultaneous loss of compressibility and direct visualization of a thrombus. Based on retrospective studies performed in patients with DVT of the lower extremities [17-19], these were classified as:

Table I. Patients' main details

Total patients enrolled	**960**
Male	675 (70%)
Female	285 (30%)
Mean age (yrs)	67.7
SD age (yrs)	10.2
CABG	624 (65%)
Valve surgery	268 (28%)
Combined CABG + valve	68 (7%)
Negative for CVC-related DVT	499 (52%)
Positive for CVC-related DVT	461 (48%)

(a) At low risk of embolism (limited) when there was only a small strip of thrombus less than 2 cm long, adhering closely to the vessel wall on one side (Figure3).

(b) At high risk of embolism when the cross-section scan showed the clot occupied at least half the lumen (subocclusive)(Figure 4a-4b) or when it appeared as an echogenic strip more than 2 cm long, attached to the wall at one end, the rest trailing freely (free-floating) (Figure 5). The US check was made on both sides.

A Doppler US of the leg veins was performed only when the patient presented the clinical criteria for lower extremity DVT or when complications suggesting or indicating PE were present.

Criteria for Diagnosis of PE

After cardiac surgery, the usual clinical manifestations of PE are often present, and any superimposed manifestations of PE become less apparent. Therefore when signs and symptoms such as dyspnea, tachypnea, hypoxia, tachycardia and hypotension were ''highly suggestive'' for PE, the diagnosis was confirmed by pulmonary angio-CT scan [20]. D-dimer levels were not utilized because high values are regularly caused by the presence of recent surgery [21].

Statistical Analysis

Preliminary statistical analysis checked the homogeneity with respect to gender and age of patients with and without CVC-related DVT and that of patients with low and high risk of embolism. Homogeneity of gender proportions was tested through the χ^2 statistic. Equality of age means was tested through the two-sample t statistic. The null hypothesis of homogeneity was never rejected, with p-values always much larger than 0.1 (see Table II-III). Similar results were also obtained with Fisher's exact test (instead of the asymptotic χ^2) and with the nonparametric Mann-Whitney U statistic (instead of the parametric two-sample t), thus reinforcing the conclusion of homogeneity of groups.

The difference in the incidences of PE in patients with CVC-related DVT was assessed through the χ^2 test and Fisher's exact test. Both methods gave remarkably similar significant results. These results provide strong evidence that the probability of PE is different if an antiplatelet is given instead of warfarin.

Results

Of the 960 eligible patients 461(48%) had an asymptomatic CVC-related DVT. Personal details (sex and age) and type of surgical interventions were similar for patients with and without a CVC-related DVT (Tables I-II). The skin condition at the point where the catheter had been inserted was unrelated to the severity of the thrombosis; only two cases, both with high-risk thrombosis, had painful swelling. A total of 159 patients with a CVCrelated DVT continued the anticoagulant therapy assigned on the basis of surgical criteria, and none of these presented clinical signs or symptoms of PE while in rehabilitation or after 3 months. Another 302 patients with a CVC-related DVT were receiving antiplatelet therapy when the US scan was performed. These were divided into two groups based on the US findings: the first group

(199 patients) consisted of those with a CVC-related DVT considered at low risk.

Table II. Comparison of the two groups, with and without CVC –related DVT

	Negative for CVC-related DVT (499)	Positive for CVC-related DVT (461)	P value
Male	339 (68%)	336 (73%)	0.9
Female	160 (32%)	125 (27%)	0.9
Mean age (years)	67.9	67.5	0.41
SD age (years)	10.1	10.4	
CABG	328(66%)	296(64%)	
Valve surgery	129(26%)	139(30%)	
CABG + valve	42 (8%)	26(6%)	

Table III. Comparison of the two groups with low and high risk of Embolism

	Low risk	High risk	P value
No.cases (total 302)	199 (66%)	103 (34%)	
Male	155 (78%)	79 (76%)	0.53
Female	44 (22%)	24 (24%)	0.53
Mean age (years)	66.7	67.2	0.7
SD age (years)	10.1	10.0	
CABG	120(60%)	70(68%)	
Valve surgery	40(21%)	21(20%)	
CABG + valve	39(19%)	12(12%)	

They continued antiplatelet therapy until the 3-month visit; this treatment could have been modified at any time if clinical reasons had arisen.

The second group comprised all those patients who were considered at high risk of embolism (103 patients). First, the antiplatelet therapy was replaced with low-molecular weight fractionated heparin as the anticoagulant until the INR was within the therapeutic range, followed by warfarin as the anticoagulant that was continued for at least 3 months or until there were no longer any US signs of thrombosis. This group had no cases of clinically manifest PE either while in hospital or at 3 months. The patients in both groups—with low or high risk of embolism—were homogeneous in both age and gender (Table III).

PE after a CVC-related DVT was seen in six cases, all belonging to first group (Figure 1). One had undergone bypass surgery and was receiving an antiplatelet agent. He complained of sudden dyspnea and bronchospasm immediately after the removal of the catheter, with an asthma-like attack requiring urgent treatment. However, this patient had no history of asthma and the hypoxemia persisting in the intensive cardiac rehabilitation unit was interpreted as a complication of PE resulting from extraction of the CVC. A Doppler US showed a free-floating thrombus in the right internal jugular (Figure5), where the catheter had been. No lower-extremity DVT was seen, but an angio-CT scan indicated emboli in both branches of the pulmonary artery(Figure6). PE was found in five other patients a few hours after their arrival from the intensive cardiosurgery unit. Three of these patients had a CABG, and were taking an antiplatelet agent, and presented with marked paroxysmal dyspnea, tachycardia, hypotension and severe hypoxemia.

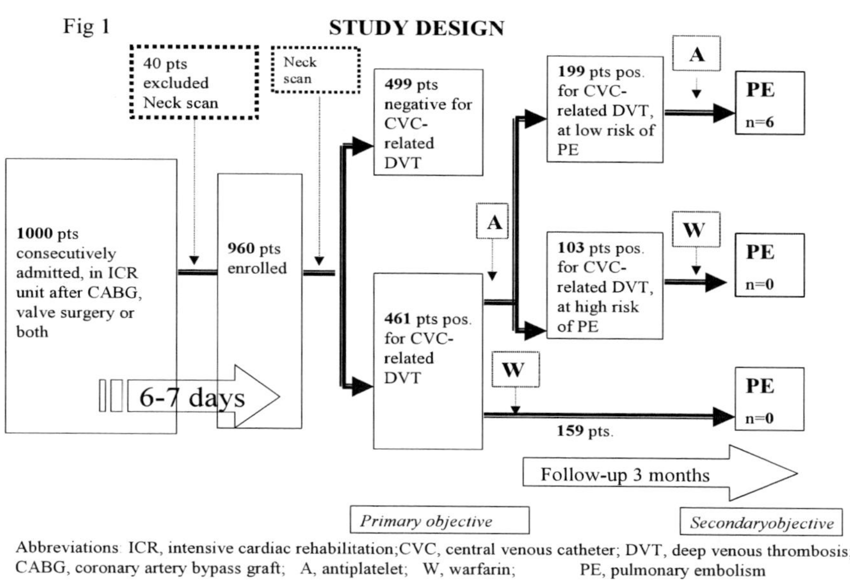

Figure 1.

All were positive for a CVC-related DVT. A pulmonary angio-CT scan found emboli in all , but none had lower-extremity DVT.

Since in one of them, the CT scan showed a PE disproportionate to the residual CVC-related DVT, US and venography of the legs, pelvic and caval areas were performed to seek other causes, but none were found.

The angio-CT scan confirmed a PE in one 54-year-old patient receiving aspirin after mitral valve repair with a ring of autologous pericardium. A DVT was found in the jugular vein, but no signs of clot were found in the lower limbs.

All patients were present at the follow-up. Internal jugular recanalization was complete in all patients with a previously thrombotic segment.

There were no deaths or symptomatic thromboembolic events between discharge and the 3-month follow-up.

The incidence of PE in patients with a CVC-related DVT who had been treated with an antiplatelet agent was 3% while in those patients given warfarin, the incidence was 0% (6/199 vs. 0/262; Figure 1). This was significant according to the χ^2 test with correction for continuity (asymptotic P value 1.6%), and by Fisher's exact test (P\0.01).

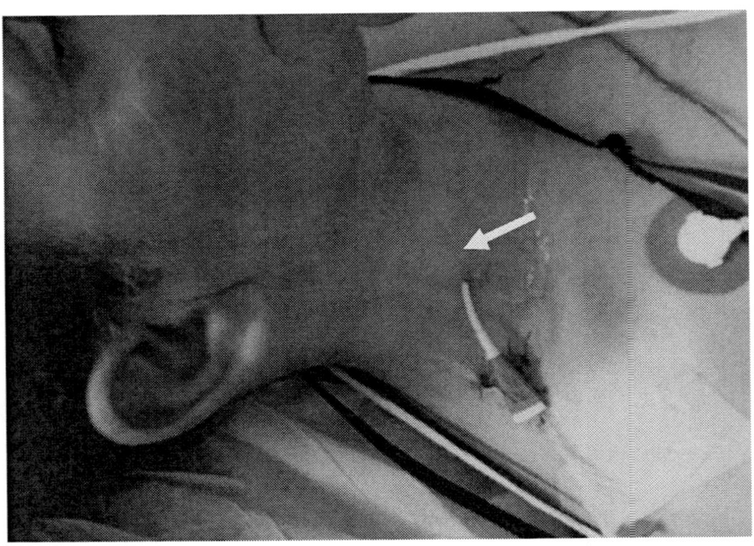

Figure 2. Central venous catheter (arrow) placet in the right internal jugular vein.

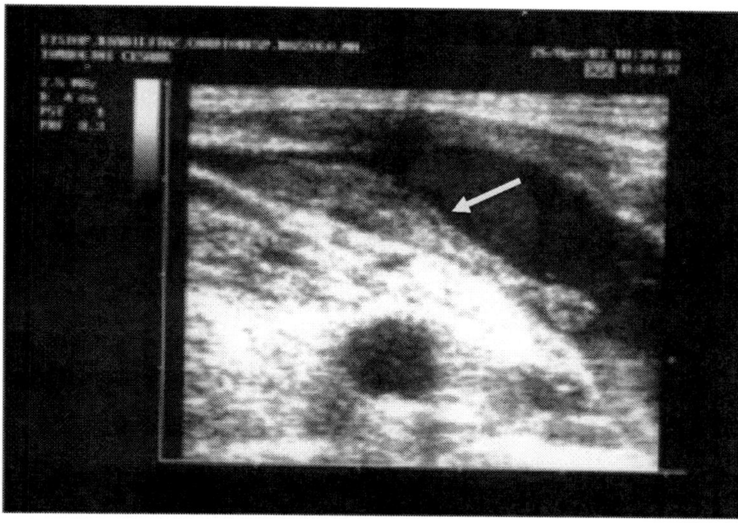

Figure 3. Limited thrombus (arrow) in the right internal jugular vein.

Discussion

About 1,200,000 heart operations are performed every year in the USA. The CVC in such cases is preferably placed in the right internal jugular vein that, according to Timsit [22], is four times more susceptible to DVT than the subclavian vein. Even so, very little is known about the prevalence of thrombotic events in these patients. In the present large series with several types of heart surgery, 48% had a DVT related to a CVC in the right internal jugular vein. This is significantly higher than the figure for lower-extremity DVT in the same type of population [23-24]. Therefore, we can assume that in the USA more than 500,000 heart operations each year may be complicated by a CVC-related DVT.

The causes or factors responsible for this complication are still not clear, just as the real reason why the thrombus forms is not known. Although catheter stiffness,number of vein punctures,the composition of solution, incorrect initial CVC positioning [25-27] or the duration of catheterization may be partial etiologic factors, a CVC in place for less than 6 days is reported to have a negligible effect on thrombus formation [28].

In the present study, patients came from various centers and had been operated on by different surgeons, so the DVT was unlikely to have been related to any particular type of catheter, or the skill in placement. In fact, the even distribution of this complication among the various centers suggests, in agreement with Joynt [29], that the real reason for CVC-related DVT is related more to the nature of the procedure than either the catheter itself or how it is applied.

These authors find no difference between heparin-impregnated and untreated catheters. Pathophysiologically,a plausible explanation is that the presence of a CVC ,as a non-biological surface in the bloodstream, activates the coagulation pathway, or induces endothelial trauma caused by the indwelling CVC or insertion procedures,or both[30].

Controversy also surrounds the question of how best to prevent a CVC-related DVT[31]. Randolph et al. [32], in their meta-analysis of 14 randomized trials, find a significant reduction in a CVC-related DVT in patients given unfractionated heparin.

In oncological patients, two multicenter trials [33-34] find that it makes no difference in prevention of a CVCrelated DVT whether or not patients take low-molecular weight heparin. On the contrary, two randomized trials [35-36] report effective prophylaxis with low-dose of warfarin or low-molecular-weight heparin.

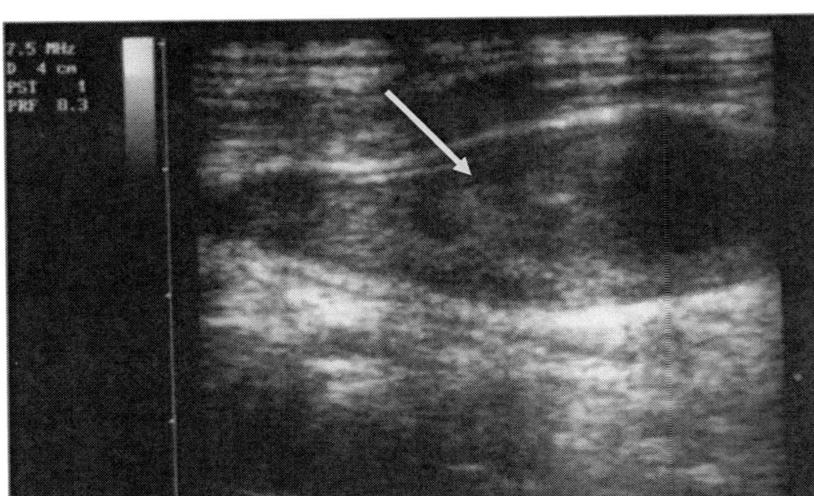

Figure 4a. Sub-occlusive (large) thrombus (arrow)in the right internal jugular vein: longitudinal section

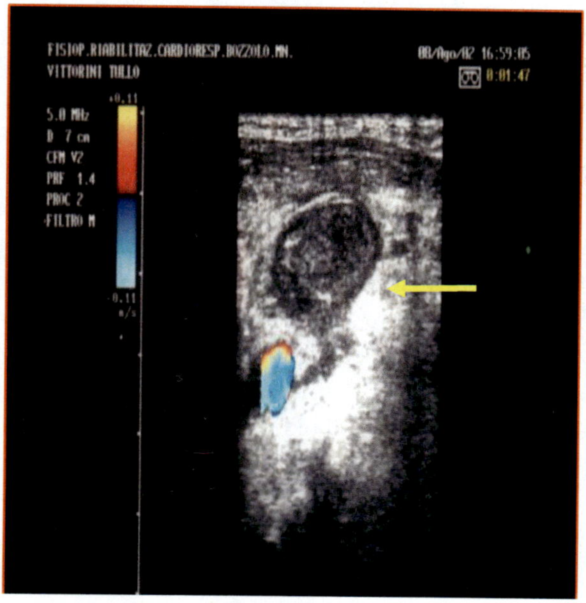

Figure 4b. Sub-occlusive (large) thrombus (arrow) in the right internal jugular vein: cross section.

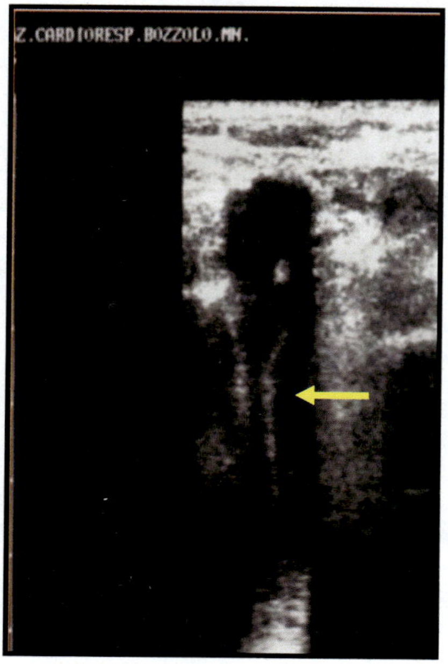

Figure 5. Free-floating thrombus(arrow) in the right internal jugular vein.

Boraks et al. [37] report a significant reduction in a CVC-related upper extremity DVT in patients with haematological malignancies given low-dose warfarin (1 mg/day), but the utility of dicoumarol (warfarin) for preventing a CVC-related DVT remains to be established [38-39].

Our findings suggest that neither heparin given during surgery nor anticoagulant therapy with heparin and warfarin immediately after surgery are very reliable for preventing venous thrombosis; moreover, early antiplatelet therapy also has no significant preventive effect. In our series, both groups were balanced according to age and gender and no concomitant role was observed on development of a CVC-related DVT or by the type of heart surgery.

As secondary endpoints, we checked for PE secondary to whether any particular pharmacological strategy reduced or prevented it. For all types of heart surgery, the literature reports an incidence of PE ranging from 0.2 to 0.9%, with a mean of 0.8%, fatal in 0.15%, referring to lower-extremity DVT [40-41]. In the arms, PE is reported in one third of patients with a CVC and DVT of an axillary, subclavian or brachiocephalic vein [42] but not the right internal jugular.

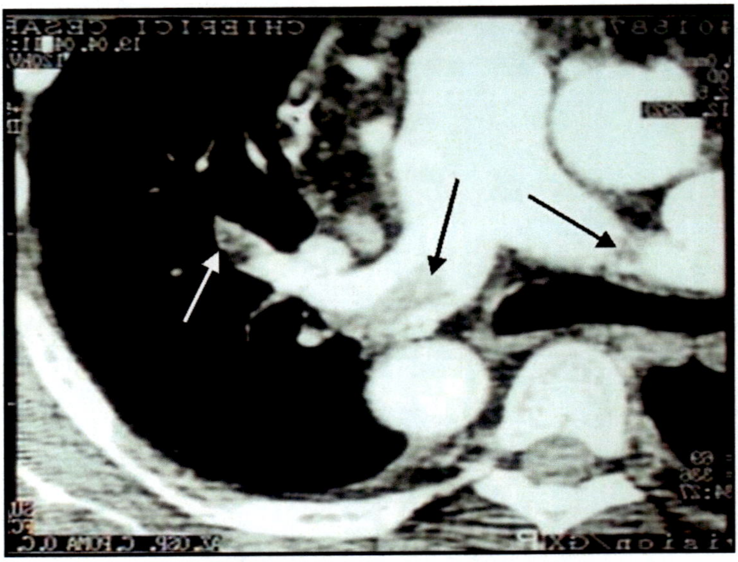

Figure 6. Angio-CT scan showing emboli in both branches of the pulmonary artery (arrows)

In our study, PE was clinically manifest in 0.6% of the whole series we studied (960 patients), a figure comparable to that reported for PE secondary to lower-extremity DVT,but incidence increase to 3% (199 patients) with catheter-related thrombosis at low risk without anticoagulant therapy (Figure1).

This, however, must be considered an underestimate because of the probability of minimal embolic events causing only non-specific symptoms, which were not interpreted as such and were more likely to be ascribed to post-operative discomfort, atelectasis, rib trauma, sternotomy or existing cardiac dysfunction.

The findings do point to one conclusion with substantial clinical relevance: though early anticoagulation with warfarin does not seem to prevent the formation of a CVC thrombus in the right internal jugular vein, it does seem to prevent clinically manifest PE in all patients with a CVC-related DVT, regardless of type of thrombus(high or low risk of embolism at US examination) or heart surgery.

Our observations coincide with Pacouret's results [43] that demonstrate that anticoagulant therapy with warfarin is able to control venous thromboembolism from proximal free floating thrombus in lower extremities without resorting to any particular prophylactic procedures.

Therefore, antiplatelet therapy alone is not only unable to prevent venous thrombosis at the site of a CVC, but also is not useful in preventing a PE. However, this finding conflicts with the meta-analysis by Antiplatelet Trialists'Collaboration [44] that used old studies and only a limited number.

Also useful as a basis for identifying CVC-related DVT patients at high or low risk of PE are morphological/ultrasonography criteria, which help establish indications for an anticoagulant rather than antiplatelet agent.

Advances in technology offer the heart surgeon new kinds of biological valve prostheses with no absolute indication for warfarin anticoagulation [45-47], so there are increasing numbers of patients who are only receiving antiplatelet therapy who might be at high risk of PE. Our findings, therefore, suggest that the proposal to reduce use of anticoagulants in prosthetic heart surgery patients is premature because surgical criteria alone are not capable of deciding on antiplatelet rather than anticoagulant therapy. In addition, sonographic screening of the CVC removal in intensive cardiosurgery unit [48] may be useful for avoiding a PE after a CVC-related DVT.

References

[1] Flinterman, LE; Van Der Meer, FJ; Rosendaal, FR; Doggen, CJ. Current perspective of venous thrombosis in the upper extremity. *J Thromb Haemost,* 2008, 6, 1262-1266.

[2] Pitter, D; Tarara, D; Wenzel, RP. Nosocomial bloodstream infection in critically ill patients: excess length of stay, extra costs, and attributable mortality. *JAMA,* 1994, 271, 1598-1601.

[3] Burns, KEA; McLaren, A. A critical review of thromboembolic complications associated with central venous catheters.*Canadian Journal of Anesthesia,* 2008, 55,532-541.

[4] Richards, MJ; Edwards, JR; Culver, DH; Gaynes, RP. Nosocomial infections in medical intensive care units in the Unites States. *Crit.Care Med.,* 1999, 27, 887-892.

[5] Merrer, J; Jonghe, B; Galliot, F. Complications of femoral and subclavian venous catheterization in critically ill patients: a randomized controlled trial. *JAMA,* 2001, 286, 700-707.

[6] McGee, DC; Gould, M. Preventing complications of central venous catheterization. *N Engl J Med,* 2003, 348, 1123-1133.

[7] Cortelezzi, A; Moia, M; Falagna, A; Pogliani, EM; Agnelli, G; Bonizzoni, E; Gussoni, G; Barbui, T; Mannucci, M. The CATHEM Study Group. Incidence of thrombotic complications in patients with haematological malignancies with central venous catheters: a prospective multicentre study. *Br J Haematol PM,* 2005, 129 (6), 811-817.

[8] Raad, I. Intravascular catheter-related infections. *Lancet,* 1998, 351, 893–898.

[9] Goldhaber, SZ; Hirsch, DR; MacDougall, RN; Polak, JF; Creager, MA; Cohn, LH. Prevention of venous thrombosis after coronary artery by-pass surgery (a randomized trial comparing two mechanical prophylaxis strategies). *Am J Cardiol,* 1995, 76, 993-996.

[10] Reis, SE; Polak, JF; Hirsch, DR; Cohn, LH; Creager, MA; Goldhaber, SZ. Frequency of deep venous thrombosis in asymptomatic patients with coronary artery bypass graft. *Am Heart J,* 1991, 122, 478-482.

[11] Ambrosetti, M; Salerno, M; Zimbelli, M; Mastropasqua, MD; Tramarin R; Pedretti RFE. Deep venous thrombosis among patients entering

cardiac rehabilitation after coronary artery bypass surgery. *Chest,* 2004, 125, 191-196.

[12] Joffe Hylton, V; Goldhaber, SZ. Upper extremity deep vein thrombosis. *Circulation,* 2002, 106, 1874-1880.

[13] Syed, M; Stein, PD; Patel, KC; Otten, TR; Holmes, R; Silbergleit, A. Upper extremity deep venous thrombosis. *Chest* 2003; 123:1953–1956

[14] Hingorani, A; Ascher, EL. Upper extremity deep venous thrombosis. *Perspective in vascular surgery and endovascular therapy,* 1999, vol.10,n.2, 47-57.

[15] Salem, DN; Stein, PD; Al-Ahmad, A; Bussey, HI; Horstkotte, D; Miller, N; Pauker, SG. Prosthetic heart valves. Bioprosthetic valves. Recommendation. In: The seventh ACCP and thrombolytic conference on antithrombotic therapy. *Chest,* 2004 , 126, 457S-482S.

[16] Geert, WH; Bergqvist, D; Pineo, GF; Heit, JA; Lassen, MR; Colwell, CW. Prevention of venous thromboembolism: general, vascular, gynecologic, urologic, laparoscopic, bariatric, thoracic and coronary artery bypass surgery. American College of Chest Physicians .Evidence based clinical practice guidelines(8th Edition). *Chest,* 2008, 133, 394S-404S.

[17] Fraser, JD; Anderson, DR. Deep venous thrombosis: recent advances and optimal investigation with US. *Radiology,* 1999 , 211, 9-24.

[18] Norris, CS; Greenfield, LJ; Hermmann, JB. Free-floating iliofemoral thrombus. A risk of pulmonary embolism. *Arch Surg,* 1985, 120 (7), 806–808.

[19] Berry, RE; George, JE; Shaver, WA. Free-floating deep venous thrombosis. A retrospective analysis. *Ann Surg,* 1990 , 6, 719-723.

[20] British Thoracic Society guidelines for the management of suspected acute pulmonary embolism. *Thorax,* 2003 , 58, 470-484.

[21] Frizzelli, R; Tortelli, O; Pinzi, C; Di Comite, V; Ghirardi, R. Contributo del D-dimer test nella diagnostica della trombosi venosa profonda del cardioperato in fase di riabilitazione intensiva. Risultati preliminari. *Ital Heart J,* 2004 , 5 (suppl.5), 126S.

[22] Timsit, JF; Farkas, JC; Boyer, JM; Martin, JB; Misset, B; Renaud, B; Carlet, J. Central vein catheter-related thrombosis in intensive care patients: incidence, risk factors and relationship with catheter-related sepsis. *Chest,* 1998 , 114, 207-213.

[23] De Laria, GA; Hunter, JA. Deep vein thrombosis. Implications after open-heart surgery. *Chest,* 1991, 99, 284-288.

[24] Gillinov, AM; Davis, EA; Alberg, AJ; Rykiel, M; Gardner, TJ; Cameron, DE. Pulmonary embolism in the cardiac surgical patient. *Ann Thorac Surg,* 1992, 5, 988-991.

[25] Stenqvist, O; Curelaru, I; Linder, LE; Gustavsoon, B. Stiffness of central venous catheters.*Acta Anaestesiologica Scandinavica,* 2008, 27, 153-157.

[26] Koksoy, C; Kuzu, A; Erden, I; Akkaya, A. The risk factors in central venous catheter-related thrombosis.*Anz Journal of Surgery,* 2008, 65, 796-798.

[27] Luciani, A; Clement, O; Halimi, P; Goudot, D; Pontier, F; Bassot, V; Luciani, JA; Avan, P; Frija, G; Bonfils, P. Catheter-related upper extremity deep venous thrombosis in cancer patients: a prospective study based on doppler US. *Radiology,* 2001, 220, 655-660.

[28] Martin, C; Viviand, X; Saux, P; Gouin, F. Upper-extremity deep vein thrombosis after central venous catheterization via the axillary vein. *Crit Care Med,* 1999 , 27, 2626-2629.

[29] Joynt, GM; Kew, J; Gomersall, CD; Leung, VJF; Liu EKH. Deep venous thrombosis caused by femoral venous catheters in critically ill adult patients. *Chest,* 2000, 117, 178-183.

[30] Blom, JW; Doggen, CJM; Osanto, S; Rosendaal, FR. Old and new risk factors for upper extremity deep venous thrombosis.*Journal of Thrombosis and Haemostasis,* 2005, 3, 2471-2478.

[31] Klerk, CP; Smorenburg, SM; Buller, HR. Thrombosis prophylaxis in patient populations with a central venous catheter.A systematic review. *Arch.Intern.Med.,* 2003, 163, 1913-1921.

[32] Randolph, AG; Cook, DJ; Calle, AG; Andrew, M. Benefit of heparin in central venous and pulmonary artery catheters. A meta-analysis of randomized controlled trials. *Chest,* 1998, 113, 165-171.

[33] Verso, M; Agnelli, G; Bertoglio, S; Di Somma, FC; Paoletti, F; Ageno, W; Bazzn, M; Parise, P; Quintavalla, R; Naglieri, E; Santoro, A; Imberti, D; Soraru, M; Mosta, S. Enoxaparin for the prevention of venous thromboembolism associated with central vein catheter; a double-blind, placebo-controlled, randomized study in cancer patients. *J Clin Oncol,* 2005, 23, 4057-4062.

[34] Karthaus, M; Kretzschmar, A; Kroning, H; Biakhov, M; Irwin, D; Marshner, N; Slabber, C; Fountzilas, G; Garin, A; Abecasis, NGF; Baronius, W; Steger, GG; Sudhoff, T; Giorgetti, C; Reichardt, P. Deltaparin for prevention of catheter-related complications in cancer patients with central venous catheters: final results of a double-blind, placebo-controlled phase III trial. *Ann Oncol,* 2006, 17, 289-296.

[35] Bern, MM; Lokich, JJ; Wallack, SR; Bothe, A; Benotti, PN; Arkin, CF; Greco, FA; Huberman, M; Moore, C. Very low doses of warfarin can prevent thrombosis in central venous catheters. *Ann Intern Med,* 1990, 112, 423-428.

[36] Mismetti, P; Mille, D; Laporte, S; Charlet, V; Buchmuller-Cordier, A; Jacquin, JP; Fournel, P; Duthrey-Dupagne, C; Deconsus, H. CIP Study Group. Low-molecular-weight heparin and very low doses of warfarin in the prevention of upper extremity thrombosis in cancer patients with indwelling long-term central venous catheter: a pilot randomized study. *Haematologica,* 2003, 88, 67-73.

[37] Boraks, P; Seale, J; Price, J; Bass, G; Ethell, M; Keeling, D; Mahendra, P; Baglin, T; Marcus, R. Prevention of central venous catheter-associated thrombosis using minidose warfarin in patients with haematological malignancies. *Br J Haematol,* 1998, 101, 483-486.

[38] Rooden, CJ; Tesselaar, M; Osanto, S; Rosendaal, FR; Huisman, MV. Deep vein thrombosis associated with central venous catheters—a review. *J Thromb Haemost,* 2005, 3, 2049-2419.

[39] Heaton, DC; Han, DY; Inder, A. Minidose (1 mg) warfarin as prophylaxis for central vein catheter thrombosis. *Intern Med J,* 2002, 32 (3), 84-88.

[40] Josa, M; Siouffi, SY; Silverman, AB; Barsamian, EM; Khuri, SF; Sharma, GV. Pulmonary embolus after cardiac surgery. *J Am Coll Cardiol,* 1993 , 21, 990-996.

[41] Shammas, NW. Pulmonary embolus after coronary artery bypass surgery: a review of the literature. *Clin Cardiol,* 2000, 23, 637-644.

[42] Prandoni, P; Polistena, P; Bernardi, E; Cogo, A; Casara, D; Verlato, F; Angelini, F; Simioni, P; Signorini, GP; Benedetti, L; Girolami, A. Upper-extremity deep vein thrombosis. Risk factors, diagnosis, and complications. *Arch Intern Med,* 1997, 157, 57-62.

[43] Pacouret, G; Alison, D; Pottier, JM; Bertrand, P; Charbonnier, B. Free-floating thrombus and embolic risk in patients with angiographically

confirmed proximal deep venous thrombosis. *Arch Intern Med*, 1997, 157, 305-308.

[44] Antiplatelet Trialists' Collaboration Collaborative overview of randomised trials of antiplatelets therapy. III: Reduction in venous thrombosis and pulmonary embolism by antiplatelet prophylaxis among surgical and medical patients. *Br Med J,* 1994, 308, 235-308.

[45] Gherli, T; Colli, A; Fragnito, C; Nicolini, F; Borrello, B; Saccani, S; D'Amico, R; Beghi, C. Comparing warfarin with aspirin after biological aortic valve replacement. A prospective study. *Circulation,* 2004, 110, 496-500.

[46] Sundt, TM; Zehr, KJ; Dearani, JA; Daly, RC; Mullany, CJ; McGregor, CGA; Puga, FJ; Orszuda, TA; Schaff, HV. Is early anticoagulation with warfarin necessary after bioprostetic aortic valve replacement? *J Thorac Cardiovasc Surg,* 2005, 129, 1024-1031.

[47] El-Husseiny, M; Salhiyyah, K; Rajia, SG; Dunning, J. Should warfarin be routinely prescribed for the first three months after a bioprosthetic valve replacement? *Interact CardioVasc Thorac Surg,* 2006, 5, 616-623.

[48] Karnik, R; Valentin, A; Winkler, WB; Donath, P; Slany, J. Duplex sonographic detection of internal jugular venous thrombosis after removal of central venous catheters. *Clin Cardiol,* 1993, 16, 26-29.

In: Cardiac Rehabilitaiton
Editor: J. T. Halliday, pp. 185-197
ISBN: 978-1-60741-918-1

Chapter VIII

Participation Compliance and Outcomes of Outpatient Cardiac Rehabilitation Programs among Women in Low Resource Settings

Nizal Sarrafzadegan and Katayoun Rabiei
Isfahan Cardiovascular Research Center,
WHO Collaborating Center for Research &
Training in Cardiovascular Disease Control,
Prevention and Rehabilitation for
Cardiac Patients in the Eastern Mediterranean Region.
Isfahan University of Medical Sciences, Isfahan, Iran

I. Cardiac Rehabilitation in Women

Cardiovascular disease (CVD) is the major cause of morbidity and mortality in women, with the vast majority of events occurred in postmenopausal age [1, 2]. Health care providers need to coordinate their efforts to effectively treat and prevent CVD in women considering their specific biology, physiology and other age related changes.

Cardiac Rehabilitation (CR), as a comprehensive approach done by multidisciplinary team, encourages and support patients to achieve and maintain optional physical and psychological health, however only a fraction of eligible patients attend and complete CR programs and women are at higher risk for underutilizing this effective preventive service [3-5].

Women attending CR programs are older [5, 6] have greater comorbidities, CVD risk factors and lower functional status than men [5]. Among CVD risk factors, hypertension and diabetes have been observed more in women [7, 8].

In recent years, quality of life is considered as one of the most important indexes used to assess the effectiveness of the treatment method undertaken for various chronic diseases including CVD. It is well documented that CR is one of the treatment modalities with satisfactory results in improving the quality of life in CVD patients [9, 10].

Women who participate in CR programs have shown rates of improvement in functional capacity and relief of anginal symptoms similar to those of men[11, 12]. Some studies have found that women may actually benefit from CR to a greater extent than men do, it might be because of greater overall improvements in women's exercise capacity [13-15].

II. Cardiac Rehabilitation in Low Resource Settings

As financial issues are considered the core component of low resource settings or low socioeconomic status (SES), therefore they have been used interchangeably. Socio-economic inequalities can be analyzed at different levels, from the individual to urban neighborhoods up to cities and whole countries. The impact of social characteristics on health in general is well established [16]. The relationship of neighborhood context and health outcomes with morbidity and mortality has added important insight into the origins of disparities in health and well-being [17] .Several studies found higher all-cause mortality in urban neighborhoods with low resource settings compared to areas with higher SES [18, 19]. This relationship is especially distinctive for mortality due to cardiovascular causes [20]. Moreover, indicators of morbidity, e.g. non- fatal ischemic heart disease (IHD) [21, 22] or self-rated poor health are also distributed disproportionately by neighborhood SES [23, 24].

IHD and it's mortality are unequally distributed between social classes, i.e. those with lower SES have greater Ischemic Heart Disease (IHD) compared with those at higher SES [25]. Hence, designing inexpensive CR centers or simplified programs for low SES patients is of special concern.

As CR has been initially established in high-income countries, its design and structure is appropriate for the SES conditions of these countries; therefore CR centers have mostly been expensive places where patients with low SES class may possibly not attend. Different countries, especially developed ones, have used various policies to resolve this problem.

In Germany, where rehabilitation is a legally-regulated sector of the health system, SES does not seem to be an important determinant for attendance and dropping out of CR programs. This issue might be explained by the fact that in Germany, CR is paid by the health insurance or pension fund in almost all cases, moreover as it is delivered as an in-patient setting, patients would have fewer problems concerning co-morbidities, transportation etc., which have been described as possible barriers to CR, particularly for those with low SES status and women[26].

Over the past years, there has been a steady increase in the number of centers providing CR in the UK, and now in this country every hospital providing treatment services for acute cardiac problems has access to CR facilities. However, 30% of ''eligible'' patients join CR programs. Groups like women, the elderly, deprived and ethnic minorities are less likely to be invited to attend or to enroll in CR programs. Home-based CR and simplified CR specific for rural areas have been designed [27].

Australia is another country perceiving this issue. Population mortality rates attributable to IHD have decreased in this country, but this did not take place to the same extent in those populations living in rural areas. Furthermore, CVD mortality rates for aboriginal Australians are twice that of other Australians, and 35% of aboriginal Australians reside in distant or inaccessible locations. Therefore, rural residents and aboriginal groups carry the greatest burden of CVD in this country. CR programs have been planned based on simplified models with less economic burden on patients and suitable for low SES settings, small cities or rural areas[28]. These programs include education, consultation and less advanced exercise protocols [29]. Some countries used other strategies to deliver CR services for low SES patients including short-term CR programs or decreasing CR sessions/week [30].

CR programs have to cover the entire society particularly those individuals with low SES levels. Based on research projects conducted in some countries, implementation of such programs were successful in increasing the patients' participation rate.

III. Factors Influencing Referral, Enrollment, Completion and Outcomes of Cardiac Rehabilitation in Women in Low Resource Settings

Despite the effectiveness of CR as a secondary prevention intervention, the majority of people who would benefit from this program may not succeed to participate in it. Successful participation in phase II of CR involves 3 distinct processes, namely referral by the physician in charge, enrollment into the program and completion of the prescribed sessions[31]. Studies examining gender differences in these processes indicate that women compared with men have a significantly lower rate of referral[32-34], are less likely to enroll[35] and have more drop out before completing phase II of CR, [32, 36].

Barriers to referral: Studies on barriers to referral to CR are limited to high-income countries, and have documented that women with less income were less likely to be referred to CR services than women with a greater annual income[6]. It is possible that these women were also uninsured or were beneficiaries of policies that did not cover CR services. Insurance coverage was found to be the strongest independent predictor of referral [34]. Race has been reported as an independent predictor of referral[37]. Patients speaking with a language other than the national one were reported to be less likely to attend CR programs largely due to communication difficulties[38].

Barriers to enrollment: One of the most powerful predictors of enrollment in CR programs is strong physician's recommendation. However primary care physicians were more likely to strongly recommend CR to men than to women [39]. The type of provider who gives follow-up care is another factor that influenced women's enrollment in CR programs [40]. The place where CR services are offered may play an important role that affect women's enrollment. Some studies revealed that compared to men, women tended to have greater participation in suburban community-based CR than in hospital-based programs [41, 42]. In addition, a direct relationship between years of education and attendance to CR programs have been suggested [43].

CR costs [44, 45], lack of insurance coverage[46], lower income level [47] and living in more deprived locations are considered among important indicators of failure to attend CR programs in women[43].

Previous studies reported that unemployed or retired patients fail to participate in CR programs more often than the employed [45-47]. Employment status is considered to be an independent predictor of enrollment in CR programs, especially among women[48-50].

Barriers to completion: Financial barriers are not only prohibiting women from enrolling in CR programs, but they lead to more drop out in those who attend as well [51].

Ethnicity is another issue that needs to be considered. A study in the US reported higher drop-out rate of black women from a CR program compared with white women, despite a greater prevalence of risk factors in the black women[52].

Employment status play different role concerning drop out in patients who attend CR programs. The odds of drop out doubled in patients who were working, opposed to those who were not working or were retired. These results suggest that the additional demands associated with work tasks and conflicts with work schedules may be the main barriers to completing CR programs [51].

Outcomes: Many studies on the gender-specific effectiveness of exercise-based CR did not document any main difference between men and women in terms of changes in medical situation, risk factors, functional capacity and quality of life [11, 12, 14, 15, 53].

IV. Opportunities for Improving Cardiac Rehabilitation among Women in Low Resource Settings

Knowledge of patient-centered, e.g. socio-demographic, psychosocial and/or clinical aspects, healthcare provider-centered, e.g., referral patterns, and program-related factors, i.e. characteristics of rehabilitation programs that are associated with women's participation and non-participation in CR, may help to identify effective strategies to improve the enrollment and completion rates of the program [3].

Gender-specific CR services are supposed to meet women's needs more than standard CR, these programs are conducted for males and females separately, and with flexibility in individualized needs and time schedule of women [54] it do not differ from standard programs primarily in the approaches being employed (e.g. cognitive-behavioral training, group discussions, health education, physical exercise).

Based on all that has been mentioned above and considering the low-income of women particularly in low resource settings and also those in religious, ethnic and racial minorities as one of the most important less-participating groups in CR programs, the following strategies can be taken into account in order to increase the participation rates of this group and their benefit from CR services:

To overcome the lack of knowledge and to improve women attitudes and beliefs toward CR programs, organizing educational sessions during hospitalization periods for patients and their families can result to increase in the participation rate in CR services. This strategy seem to be effective even for minorities, low SES and low-educated women as both health care providers and family members play their roles in providing the information of the importance of CR programs [55]. The establishment of proper relationship between patients and hospital's personnel during the hospitalization period seems to be an important key issue as well. This communication may induce positive attitudes towards CR programs [52].

Another suggested strategy is the establishment of community or health centers-based CR programs that are suitable for rural areas or areas that have hospitals without phase II CR facilities [56].

Although positive outcomes were found with telephone contacts and home visits [57] that may fit women needs and preferences, however, because of financial limitations, this strategy is not suggested for women living in low resource settings.

Automatic referral to CR and secondary prevention services for every eligible patient based on AACVPR/ACC/AHA 2007 guidelines is another strategy that may increase the enrolment of women in CR programs [58].In this case insurance reimbursement for participation is needed.

Some studies have reported nonsuccessful outcomes from home-based CR programs in women mainly due to lower exercise adherence [59]. However, home-based CR programs offer a flexible and feasible method particularly for women of older age, those with time constraints and numerous responsibilities or those who have social inhibition to increase their participation rate.

Conclusion

In general, although women benefit similar to men from CR programs, however, they have significant lower rate of referral, enrollment and completing the whole program. This is more likely to happen in low SES groups or women living in low resource settings. Pre-discharge educational sessions for patients and their families, improving the communication between patients and health professionals, community and home-based CR programs, automatic referral system to CR and insurance coverage seem to be helpful. Specific, flexible CR programs for women based on their psychological conditions, familial roles, cultural and social as well as economic status are good opportunities for improving CR among women specifically those who live in low resource settings.

References

[1] Heart and stroke statistical update. Dallas, Texas: *American Heart association*. 2000.

[2] Menopause and risk factors for coronary heart disease. *N Engl Jour Med.*, 1989, 321, 641-646.

[3] Scott, LA; Ben-Or, K; Allen, JK. Why are women missing from outpatient cardiac rehabilitation programs? A review of multilevel

factors affecting referral, enrollment, and completion. *Journal of women's health*, (2002). 2002 Nov; 11(9), 773-91.

[4] Bittner, V; Sanderson, BK. Women in cardiac rehabilitation. *Journal of the American Medical Women's Association*, (1972). 2003, Fall; 58(4), 227-35.

[5] Thomas, RJ; Miller, NH; Lamendola, C; Berra, K; Hedback, B; Durstine, JL; Haskell, W. National Survey on Gender Differences in Cardiac Rehabilitation Programs. Patient characteristics and enrollment patterns. *Journal of cardiopulmonary rehabilitation.*, 1996, Nov-Dec; 16(6), 402-12.

[6] Allen, JK; Scott, LB; Stewart, KJ; Young, DR. Disparities in women's referral to and enrollment in outpatient cardiac rehabilitation. *Journal of general internal medicine.*, 2004, Jul; 19(7), 747-53.

[7] Cannistra, LB; Balady, GJ; O'Malley, CJ; Weiner, DA; Ryan, TJ. Comparison of the clinical profile and outcome of women and men in cardiac rehabilitation. *Am J Cardiol.*, 1992 May 15, 69(16), 1274-9

[8] Sanderson, BK; Bittner, V. Women in cardiac rehabilitation: outcomes and identifying risk for dropout. *American heart journal.*, 2005, Nov; 150(5), 1052-8.

[9] Brown, N; Melville, M; Gray, D; Young, T; Munro, J; Skene, AM; Hampton JR. Quality of life four years after acute myocardial infarction: short form 36 scores compared with a normal population. *Heart (British Cardiac Society).*, 1999, Apr;81(4), 352-8.

[10] Gardner, JK; McConnell, TR; Klinger, TA; Herman, CP; Hauck, CA; Laubach Jr CA. Quality of life and self-efficacy: gender and diagnoses considerations for management during cardiac rehabilitation. *Journal of cardiopulmonary rehabilitation.*, 2003, Jul-Aug;23(4), 299-306.

[11] Cannistra, LB; Balady, GJ; O'Malley, CJ; Weiner, DA; Ryan, TJ. Comparison of the clinical profile and outcome of women and men in cardiac rehabilitation. *The American journal of cardiology.*, 1992, May 15, 69(16), 1274-9.

[12] Sarrafzadegan, N; Rabiei, K; Kabir, A; Sadeghi, M; Khosravi, A; Asgari, S; Taghipour, HR; Roohafza, H. Gender differences in risk factors and outcomes after cardiac rehabilitation. *Acta cardiologica.*, 2008, Dec; 63(6), 763-70.

[13] Lavie, CJ; Milani, RV. Effects of cardiac rehabilitation and exercise training on exercise capacity, coronary risk factors, behavioral

characteristics, and quality of life in women. *The American journal of cardiology.*, 1995, Feb 15, 75(5), 340-3.

[14] Kennedy, MD; Haykowsky, M; Daub, B; Van Lohuizen, K; Knapik, G; Black B. Effects of a comprehensive cardiac rehabilitation program on quality of life and exercise tolerance in women: A retrospective analysis. *Current controlled trials in cardiovascular medicine.*, 2003, Apr 1, 4(1), 1.

[15] Verrill, D; Barton, C; Beasley, W; Brennan, M; Lippard, M; King, C. Quality of life measures and gender comparisons in North Carolina Cardiac Rehabilitation Programs. *Journal of cardiopulmonary rehabilitation.*, 2001, Jan-Feb, 21(1), 37-46.

[16] Marmot, M; Wilkinson, RG. Social deterninants of health 2nd edition. Oxford: *Oxford University Press*; 2006.

[17] van Lenthe, FJ. Aggregate deprivation and effects on health. In Social inequalities in health Edited by: Siegrist J, Marmot M. Oxford: *Oxford University Press*, 2006, 167-192.

[18] Martikainen, P; Kauppinen, TM; Valkonen, T. Effects of the characteristics of neighbourhoods and the characteristics of people on cause specific mortality: a register based follow up study of 252,000 men. *J Epidemiol Community Health*, 2003, 57, 210-217.

[19] Bosma, H; van de Mheen, HD; Borsboom, GJ; Mackenbach, JP. Neighborhood socioeconomic status and all-cause mortality. *Am J Epidemiol*, 2001, 153, 363-371.

[20] Macintyre, K; Stewart, S; Chalmer, J; Pell, J; Finlayson, A; Boyd, J; Redpath, A; McMurray, J; Capewell, S. Relation between socioeconomic deprivation and death from a first myocardial infarction in Scotland: population based analysis. *BMJ*, 2001, 322, 1152-1153.

[21] Diez Roux, AV; Merkin, SS; Arnett, D; Chambless, L; Massing, M; Nieto, FJ; Sorlie, P; Szklo, M; Tyroler, HA; Watson, RL. Neighborhood of residence and incidence of coronary heart disease. *N Engl J Med*, 2001, 345, 99-106.

[22] Winkleby, M; Sundquist, K; Cubbin, C. Inequities in CHD incidence and case fatality by neighborhood deprivation. *Am J of Prev Med*, 2007, 32, 97-106.

[23] Reijneveld, SA. Neighbourhood socioeconomic context and self reported health and smoking: a secondary analysis of data on seven cities. *J Epidemiol Community Health*, 2002, 56, 935-942.

[24] Stafford, M; Martikainen, P; Lahelma, E; Marmot, M. Neighbourhoods and self rated health: a comparison of public sector employees in London and Helsinki. *J Epidemiol Community Health*, 2004, 58, 772-778.

[25] Hemmingsson, T; Lundberg, I. How far are socioeconomic differences in coronary heart disease hospitalization, all-cause mortality and cardiovascular mortality among adult Swedish males attributable to negative childhood circumstances and behaviour in adolescence? *International journal of epidemiology*., 2005, Apr, 34(2), 260-7.

[26] Karoff, M; Held, K; Bjarnason-Wehrens, B.Cardiac rehabilitation in Germany. *Eur J Cardiovasc Prev Rehabil*., 2007, Feb, 14(1), 18-27

[27] Bethell, H; Lewin, R; Dalal. H. Cardiac rehabilitation in the United Kingdom.*Heart*, 2009, 95, 271-275

[28] Joanne Dollard , JS; David, R. Thompson Simon Stewart. Broadening the reach of cardiac rehabilitation to rural and remote Australia. *European Journal of Cardiovascular Nursing*., 2004, 3 27–42.

[29] Acute Coronary Syndrome Guidelines Working Group. Guidelines for the management of acute coronary syndromes, 2006. *Med J Aust*, 2006, 184, (8 Suppl): S1-S32.

[30] Vanhees, L; McGee, HM; Dugmore, LD; et al. The Carinex Survey: current guidelines and practices in cardiacrehabilitation in Europe. *Belgium: Acco, Leuven*, 1999.

[31] Parkosewich, JA. Cardiac rehabilitation barriers and opportunities among women with cardiovascular disease. *Cardiology in review*., 2008, Jan-Feb, 16(1), 36-52.

[32] Caulin-Glaser, T; Blum, M; Schmeizl, R; Prigerson, HG; Zaret, B; Mazure, CM. Gender differences in referral to cardiac rehabilitation programs after revascularization. *Journal of cardiopulmonary rehabilitation*., 2001, Jan-Feb, 21(1), 24-30.

[33] Halm, M; Penque, S; Doll, N; Beahrs, M. Women and cardiac rehabilitation: referral and compliance patterns. *The Journal of cardiovascular nursing*., 1999, Apr, 13(3), 83-92.

[34] Bongard, V; Grenier, O; Ferrieres, J; Danchin, N; Cantet, C; Amelineau, E; Cambou, JP. Drug prescriptions and referral to cardiac rehabilitation after acute coronary events: comparison between men and women in the French PREVENIR Survey. *International journal of cardiology*., 2004, Feb; 93(2-3), 217-23.

[35] Lieberman, L; Meana, M; Stewart, D. Cardiac rehabilitation: gender differences in factors influencing participation. *Journal of women's health / the official publication of the Society for the Advancement of Women's Health Research.*, 1998 Aug;7(6), 717-23.

[36] Yohannes, AM; Yalfani, A; Doherty, P; Bundy, C. Predictors of drop-out from an outpatient cardiac rehabilitation programme. *Clinical rehabilitation.*, 2007, Mar; 21(3), 222-9.

[37] Bittner, V; Sanderson, B; Breland, J; Green, D. Referral patterns to a University-based cardiac rehabilitation program. *The American journal of cardiology.*, 1999, Jan 15, 83(2), 252-5, A5.

[38] Cortes, O; Arthur, HM. Determinants of referral to cardiac rehabilitation programs in patients with coronary artery disease: a systematic review. *American heart journal.*, 2006, Feb; 151(2), 249-56.

[39] Ades, PA; Waldmann, ML; Polk, DM; Coflesky JT. Referral patterns and exercise response in the rehabilitation of female coronary patients aged greater than or equal to 62 years. *The American journal of cardiology.*, 1992, Jun 1, 69(17), 1422-5.

[40] Barber, K; Stommel, M; Kroll, J; Holmes-Rovner, M; McIntosh, B. Cardiac rehabilitation for community-based patients with myocardial infarction: factors predicting discharge recommendation and participation. *Journal of clinical epidemiology.*, 2001, Oct; 54(10), 1025-30.

[41] Blackburn, GG; Foody, JM; Sprecher, DL; Park, E; Apperson-Hansen C; Pashkow FJ. Cardiac rehabilitation participation patterns in a large, tertiary care center: evidence for selection bias. *Journal of cardiopulmonary rehabilitation.*, 2000, May-Jun;20(3), 189-95.

[42] Filip, J; McGillen, C; Mosca, L. Patient preferences for cardiac rehabilitation and desired program elements. *Journal of cardiopulmonary rehabilitation.*, 1999, Nov-Dec;19(6), 339-43.

[43] Harlan, WR; 3rd, Sandler, SA; Lee, KL; Lam, LC; Mark, DB. Importance of baseline functional and socioeconomic factors for participation in cardiac rehabilitation. *The American journal of cardiology.*, 1995, Jul 1, 76(1), 36-9.

[44] Heid, HG; Schmelzer, M. Influences on women's participation in cardiac rehabilitation. *Rehabil Nurs.*, 2004, Jul-Aug; 29(4), 116-21.

[45] Grace, SL; Abbey, SE; Shnek, ZM; Irvine, J; Franche, RL; Stewart, DE. Cardiac rehabilitation II: referral and participation. *General hospital psychiatry.*, 2002, May-Jun;24(3), 127-34.

[46] Mochari, H; Lee, JR; Kligfield, P; Mosca, L. Ethnic differences in barriers and referral to cardiac rehabilitation among women hospitalized with coronary heart disease. *Preventive cardiology.*, 2006, Winter, 9(1), 8-13.

[47] Husak, L; Krumholz, HM; Lin, ZQ; Kasl, SV; Mattera, JA; Roumanis SA; Vaccarino V. Social support as a predictor of participation in cardiac rehabilitation after coronary artery bypass graft surgery. *Journal of cardiopulmonary rehabilitation.*, 2004, Jan-Feb;24(1), 19-26.

[48] Gallagher, R; McKinley, S; Dracup, K. Predictors of women's attendance at cardiac rehabilitation programs. *Progress in cardiovascular nursing.*, 2003, Summer, 18(3), 121-6.

[49] Evenson, KR; Rosamond, WD; Luepker, RV. Predictors of outpatient cardiac rehabilitation utilization: the Minnesota Heart Surgery Registry. *Journal of cardiopulmonary rehabilitation.*, 1998, May-Jun;18(3), 192-8.

[50] Lane, D; Carroll, D; Ring, C; Beevers, DG; Lip, GY. Predictors of attendance at cardiac rehabilitation after myocardial infarction. *Journal of psychosomatic research.*, 2001, Sep;51(3), 497-501.

[51] Sanderson, BK; Phillips, MM; Gerald, L; DiLillo, V; Bittner, V. Factors associated with the failure of patients to complete cardiac rehabilitation for medical and nonmedical reasons. *Journal of cardiopulmonary rehabilitation.*, 2003, Jul-Aug, 23(4), 281-9.

[52] Cannistra, LB; O'Malley, CJ; Balady, GJ. Comparison of outcome of cardiac rehabilitation in black women and white women. *The American journal of cardiology.*, 1995 May 1;75(14), 890-3.

[53] Todaro, JF; Shen, BJ; Niaura, R; Tilkemeier, PL; Roberts, BH. Do men and women achieve similar benefits from cardiac rehabilitation? *Journal of cardiopulmonary rehabilitation.*, 2004, Jan-Feb, 24(1), 45-51.

[54] Sarrafzadegan, N; Rabiei, K; Shirani, S; Kabir, A; Mohammadifard, N; Roohafza, H. Drop-out predictors in cardiac rehabilitation programmes and the impact of sex differences among coronary heart disease patients in an Iranian sample: a cohort study. *Clinical rehabilitation.*, 2007, Apr; 21(4), 362-72.

[55] King, KM; Humen, DP; Smith, HL; Phan, CL; Teo, KK. Predicting and explaining cardiac rehabilitation attendance. *The Canadian journal of cardiology.*, 2001, Mar; 17(3), 291-6.

[56] Carroll, DL. Capacity for direct attention in patients undergoing percutaneous coronary intervention: the effects of psychological distress. *Progress in cardiovascular nursing.*, 2005, Winter; 20(1), 11-6.

[57] Lewin, B; Robertson, IH; Cay, EL; Irving, JB; Campbell, M. Effects of self-help post-myocardial-infarction rehabilitation on psychological adjustment and use of health services. *Lancet.*, 1992, Apr 25, 339(8800), 1036-40.

[58] Fischer, JP. Automatic referral to cardiac rehabilitation. *The Journal of cardiovascular nursing.*, 2008, Nov-Dec; 23(6), 474-9.

[59] Jolly, K; Taylor, R; Lip, GY; Greenfield, S; Raftery, J; Mant, J; Lane, D; Jones, M; Lee, KW; Stevens, A. The Birmingham Rehabilitation Uptake Maximisation Study (BRUM). Home-based compared with hospital-based cardiac rehabilitation in a multi-ethnic population: cost-effectiveness and patient adherence. *Health technology assessment (Winchester, England).* 2007, Sep;11(35), 1-118.

In: Cardiac Rehabilitaiton
Editor: J. T. Halliday, pp. 199-210
ISBN: 978-1-60741-918-1

Chapter IX

Diagnosis and Treatment of Depression and Anxiety in Patients in Cardiac Rehabilitation

Karl Kristjánsson, Þórunn Guðmundsdóttir and Magnús R Jónasson
Reykjalundur Rehabilitation Center 270 Mosfellsbær Iceland

Abstract

Objective

The aim of this study was to estimate the prevalence of depression and anxiety among patients in cardiac rehabilitation at Reykjalundur Rehabilitation Center and to study the impact of a 4-5 weeks inpatient cardiac rehabilitation program on these symptoms. Secondly we wished to compare the concordance of our clinical diagnosis with the results of a standardized psychometric scale, Hospital Anxiety and Depression scale, HAD.

Materials and Methods

Of 224 patients in one year, 200 (89.3%) were included in the study, 151 men and 49 women. The patients were first evaluated by a doctor and a nurse separately at the arrival and a clinical evaluation was made jointly. Shortly after arrival and before departure a HAD questionnaire was to be answered. All new psychiatric treatment was recorded.

Results

Prevalence of depression as measured by HAD was reduced from 9.5% to 3.1% and anxiety from 11.6% to 2.5%. The sensitivity of clinical diagnosis of depression as compared to the results of HAD was 73.7% and specificity 87.3%. For anxiety the sensitivity was 86.4% and specificity was 79.2%. The predictive value of a positive clinical diagnosis of depressions was 37.8% and anxiety 33.9%, but predictive value of a negative clinical diagnosis was 96.9% and anxiety 97.9% respectively.

Conclusion

The prevalence of depression and anxiety is similar or somewhat lower than in other studies on patients with cardiac diseases. The agreement of clinical diagnosis and HAD questionnaire was acceptable and the questionnaire will not be used routinely. A comprehensive cardiac rehabilitation program seems to substantially reduce symptoms of depression and anxiety among patients in cardiac rehabilitation at Reykjalundur.

Introduction

Epidemiological research has strongly indicated that depression is an independent risk factor for coronary diseases [1]. Depression often follows coronary diseases and depressed cardiac patients have increased risk of suffering from new infarction and their death rate is higher [2]. The prevalence of depression among patients with coronary disease differs considerably from one study to another. It can be estimated that up to one third of the patients will get depressed after myocardial infarction [3]. It is also well known that depressed coronary patients tend to seek more frequently to their doctors and to emergency rooms and are more frequently hospitalized compared to those not depressed [2]. It is therefore important to diagnose depression among cardiac patients but that can be somewhat difficult. Depressed cardiac patients are often preoccupied by their somatic symptoms and some of their symptoms can be of both physical and psychological origin such as tiredness, lack of condition and initiative. It is well known that depression is frequently under-diagnosed among patients with coronary heart disease [3]. Epidemiological studies have similarly shown that patients with anxiety symptoms are more prone to die from coronary heart diseases [4, 5].

The purpose of this study was to estimate the prevalence of depression and anxiety with those patients that were admitted to the cardiac rehabilitation program at Reykjalundur, Rehabilitation Center, Iceland. At the same time we wanted to compare the concordance of clinical diagnosis and the results of an established depression and anxiety psychometric scale to evaluate the need to systematically screen all patients for depression and anxiety. Finally, we wanted to evaluate the effect of a comprehensive cardiac rehabilitation program on symptoms of depression and anxiety among the patients both at the beginning and at the end of the program.

Material and Methods

A comprehensive inpatient cardiac rehabilitation program has been running continuously at Reykjalundur Rehabilitation Center since 1982. The main reasons for admission of patients to the cardiac rehabilitation are physical exercise and adaption after coronary artery bypass surgery, myocardial infarction and percutaneus angioplasty. To some extent there are also patients who have not had recent cardiac events but need to change their lifestyle and reduce risk factors. The main emphasis has been on increasing strength and endurance, lifestyle modification and patient education. Approximately 50% of the patients are at the same time offered participation in a patient work-shop on balanced daily life, relaxation and stress-management as part of the cardiac rehabilitation program. To this work-shop there have mostly been invited younger people dealing with stress situations and unequal distribution between time spent on work vs. free time and family relations. The usual time spent on the treatment is 4-6 weeks.

For the study we used The Hospital Anxiety and Depression Scale questionnaire (HAD) [6], which is designed to screen for depression and anxiety among patients with physical illnesses. This scale has been widely used previously in similar studies [7-9]. All patients who came into the cardiac rehabilitation program at Reykjalundur from April 1st 2005 to March 31st 2006 were invited to participate in the study. Over this time period 224 patients came to the clinic and 200 (89.3%) of them agreed to take part. Of those 24 individuals who did not participate, 10 did not sign the agreement, 7 did not return all of the questionnaires, 3 did not finish the program and 4 were excluded for other reasons. All necessary permissions for the study were obtained from The National Bioethics Committee and The Data Protection Authority.

At the start of the rehabilitation the doctors and nurses separately evaluated the patients for clinical depression and/or anxiety and if so to what extent. Their clinical condition was rated in three categories, not – probably – depressed/anxious both for anxiety and depression. This evaluation is in accordance with the HAD scoring system, where 0-7 points are normal, 8-10 are probable and 11 points or more are an indication of depression/anxiety. The doctors and nurses then compared their ratings, which were made separately and recorded the results. If they did not agree in their evaluation, the one that rated higher was registered. A special note was made if the patient had been previously diagnosed with depression or anxiety. The HAD questionnaires were filled out by the patients both in the beginning and at the end of the treatment program.

Treatment routines for psychiatric illnesses were not changed during the study period from what they had been previously. At discharge we recorded all new treatment for depression/anxiety.

Statistics

Values are shown as averages with one standard deviation, SD. Comparison of groups was done with chi-square tests but comparison of depression and anxiety according to HAD scale as a continuous value, but as the variables were not with normal distribution, non-parametric tests were used with Wilcoxon matched-pairs signed-ranks test. To study the correlation between depression and anxiety scores from the HAD questionnaire and age we used the Spearman rank correlation. The statistic package that was used was GraphPad InStat version 3.05.

Results

Of 200 participants in the study there were 151 men and 49 women. Mean age among the male was 61.7 years (SD 10.8) but the female were 62.7 years (SD 10.1). Most of the patients came after coronary artery bypass surgery or other coronary events or symptoms. Few came because of other cardiac diseases, such as heart failure and cardiac valve replacement. (Table I).

Table I. Number of patients by gender and after indication for cardiac rehabilitation

	Male	Female	Total	Ratio of the total patient material
Coronary artery bypass surgery	78	18	96	48,0 %
Myocardial infarction	24	10	34	17,0 %
Op mitral/aortic valve	12	6	18	9,0 %
Chronic ischemic heart disease	12	4	16	8,0 %
Percutaneus angioplasty	13	3	16	8,0 %
Heart failure	6	2	8	4,0 %
Cardiac arrythmias	2	1	3	1,5 %
Other indications	4	5	9	4,5 %
Total	151	49	200	100 %

Among the patients 39 had previous history of depression and 23 had previously been diagnosed with anxiety. After clinical interviews at admission 37 were diagnosed as depressed (18.5%) but 19 (9.5%) according to the results of HAD questionnaire. Similarly 56 were clinically diagnosed with anxiety (28.0%) but 22 (11%) had anxiety according to HAD. No significant difference was found in the incidence of depression or anxiety between men and women whether based on previous history, clinical diagnosis or results from the HAD (Table II). There was no significant correlation between age and depression on HAD, Spearman $r = 0.0012$, $p = 0.986$, but on the other hand there was a quite strong negative correlation between age and anxiety on HAD, $r = -0.22$, $p = 0.0014$, that is, there was more anxiety among younger patients. There was a rather little overlap between the group that had previous history of depression and anxiety and the group that fulfilled the positive screening criteria according to HAD at arrival (Figure 1). It can therefore be concluded that a substantial part of the symptoms at arrival were new and had not been diagnosed previously.

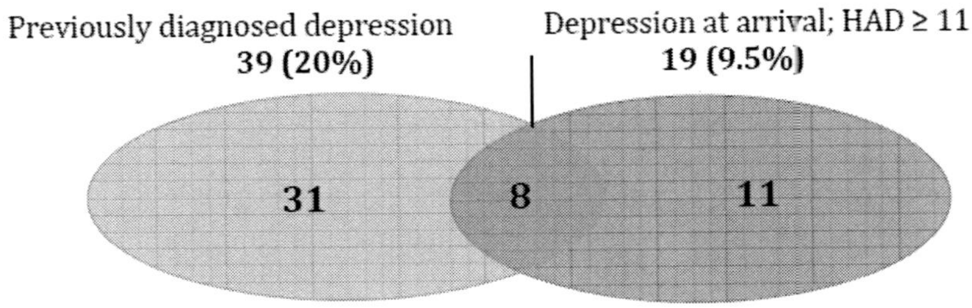

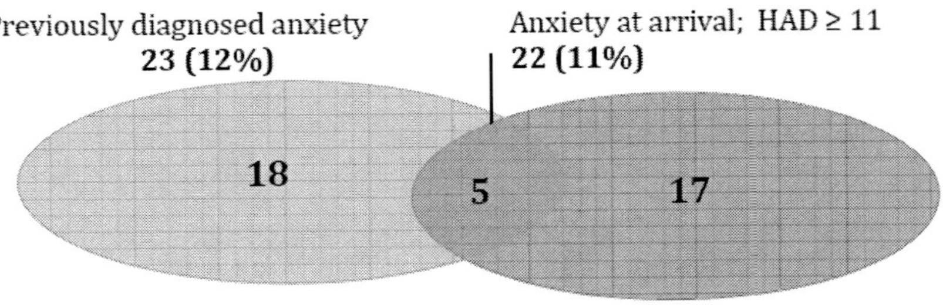

Figure I. Overlap between previously diagnosed depression/anxiety and depression/anxiety at arrival, with HAD ≥ 11.

Of those 200 patients 87 attended patient information sessions on balancing daily living. In addition to the usual cardiac rehabilitation the patients were treated for psychiatric problems as needed. Nine patients were treated by a psychiatric consultant, three by psychologist, fourteen got antidepressive medication, eighteen anxiolytic medication and five cognitive behavioral therapy.

In order to evaluate the change in psychiatric symptoms during the treatment period the results from the HAD tests both at arrival and departure were compared. We examined both the number of patients that fulfilled the positive screening criteria (HAD $\geq$ 11) at each time and we also compared the HAD results as a continuous variable.

The prevalence of depression and anxiety turned out to be much lower at the end of the program than at the beginning, the prevalence of depression was diminished from 9.5% to 3% or by 72% and the prevalence of anxiety was similarly reduced from 11.0% to 2.5% or 77% (Table III).

When the results from the HAD questionnaire were compared as continuous variables the average value for depression was reduced from 4.79 to 3.61 (paired Wilcoxon test $p < 0.0001$) and the average value from HAD for anxiety was reduced from 4.66 to 3.30 ($p < 0.0001$).

Table II. Comparison on the prevalence of depression/anxiety among men and women at admittance

	Male		**Female**		**Total**		
	N=151	**%**	**N=49**	**%**	**N=200**	**%**	**p-value**
Previous history of depression	29	*19,2%*	10	*20,4%*	39	*19,5%*	0,85
Previous history of anxiety	17	*11,3%*	6	*12,2%*	23	*11,5%*	0,85
Depression, clinical diagnosis	24	*15,9%*	13	*26,5%*	37	*18,5%*	0,15
Anxiety, clinical diagnosis	40	*26,5%*	16	*32,7%*	56	*28,0%*	0,51
Depression HAD $\geq$11	15	*9,9%*	4	*8,2%*	19	*9,5%*	0,93
Anxiety HAD $\geq$11	15	*9,9%*	7	*14,3%*	22	*11,0%*	0,56

There was a strong correlation between depression and anxiety, 11 patients were positive both on the depression and anxiety scale at arrival. Those who were both depressed and anxious had an average score of 14.1 at arrival but 7.9 at departure. Those who were depressed but not anxious had an average score of 11.7 at arrival but 6.25 at departure. The relative reduction of symptoms is therefore similar and more severe and widespread symptoms at the start do not seem to stay in the way of a good recovery.

To assess the sensitivity of clinical evaluation by the doctors and nurses at the patient interview the results of the clinical diagnosis after arrival were compared to the frequency of depression/anxiety according to the results from the HAD questionnaires. The sensitivity and specificity of the clinical diagnosis for both depression and anxiety seem to be quite acceptable but the predictive value of positive clinical diagnosis was much lower. The predictive value of negative clinical diagnosis was on the other hand high or 97-98% (Table IV).

Table III. Prevalence of depression and anxiety, as measured by HAD questionnaire at admittance and discharge of cardiac rehabilitation at Reykjalundur.

	Depression				Anxiety			
	Admittance		Discharge		Admittance		Discharge	
Yes	19	*9,5%*	6	*3,0%*	22	*11,0%*	5	*2,5%*
Possible	27	*13,5%*	12	*6,0%*	26	*13,0%*	16	*8,0%*
No	154	*77,0%*	182	*91,0%*	152	*76,0%*	179	*89,5%*

Table IV. Sensitivity, specificity and predictive value of positive/negative clinical diagnosis of depression and anxiety.

	Depression	**Anxiety**
Sensitivity	73,7%	86,4%
Specificity	87,3%	79,2%
Predictive value of positive clinical diagnosis	37,8%	33,9%
Predictive value of negative clinical diagnosis	96,9%	97,9%

Discussion

This study, which included a large part of the patients that came for cardiac rehabilitation at Reykjalundur Rehabilitation Center over a one-year period, revealed that depression and anxiety was a common problem at arrival. At discharge from the program those symptoms were substantially reduced. Most of those who where diagnosed depressed or anxious on the HAD screening at arrival were diagnosed similarly during the routine interviews with doctors and nurses at arrival. The sensitivity and specificity was quite good, but the doctors and nurses shared evaluation had a tendency to over-diagnose depression and anxiety compared to HAD.

The prevalence of depression and anxiety among cardiac patients varies by which tests and diagnostic limits are used or from 17-28% [3,10]. The prevalence of depression and anxiety among those who came for cardiac rehabilitation at Reykjalundur seems to be comparable or somewhat lower, but the comparison is difficult as the studies have a different design. A screening for psychiatric disorders done in a population study in Iceland 2002 showed the prevalence to be 17.5%, but if those treated with medication for psychiatric disorders were added the prevalence was further increased to 20.7% [11].

Anxiety, anger and hostility have been shown to be more prevalent among younger cardiac patients, but depression is less dependent on age [10]. In our study anxiety was also more frequent among younger patients but depression was more evenly distributed in all age groups. It is therefore reasonable to conclude that a participation in a patient workshop on balanced daily life, relaxation and stress-management can be particularly useful for the younger patients. Other studies have shown higher rates of psychiatric disturbances among women, particularly anxiety[12]. Our results did however not show any statistical differences between men and women but as the number of women where only a quarter of the total number of patients, a statistical difference in a subgroup can be difficult to distinguish.

One of the main aims for this study was to evaluate how successful we are in diagnosing common psychiatric illnesses like depression and anxiety in our routine interviews at admittance to the cardiac rehabilitation. We therefore tried to remain with the ordinary work procedures in patient interviews on arrival and staff meetings. The results of the study show that standard admittance interviews were quite effective when it came to spotting psychiatric problems. From the data of this study we therefore concluded that the gain of a routine screening of all patients would not justify the cost and extra work that the use of the HAD questionnaire would involve. There are no absolute rules as to when screening tests are justified but it has to be considered if the usual clinical procedures result in considerable missing of cases and at what consequences. In this particular situation the sensitivity of the diagnosis was acceptable and the psychiatric symptoms that were prevalent at arrival were reduced substantially in the routine treatment. The usefulness of HAD questionnaires does therefore seem to be mostly in screening of patients where depression or anxiety is suspected. Another gain by using questionnaires both at the beginning and end of the treatment period is that it can give a numerical value for the effect of the treatment. It is clear that one can not rely on screening tools like HAD alone in diagnosing psychiatric illnesses among those patients and we will therefore continue to need good clinical examination in the future.

The main strength of this study was a high participation rate among the patients that came for rehabilitation during the study period and that the same group of staff did the examinations and evaluations of the patients throughout the study period. As the same questionnaires were used by all participants, both at the start and by the end of the treatment we could also assess the results on the anxiety and depressive symptoms during the treatment period. The main weakness of the study was that we did not have a comparison group that would have been left untreated, but for various reasons that would have been difficult to do. Depression after being diagnosed with a cardiac illness can be resistant and it does not always subside spontaneously without treatment [3]. From this study we can not fully clarify what elements of the rehabilitations program were most effective in enhancing the psychiatric health to the degree that we observed. However as only a few of the patients got a specific psychiatric treatment or antidepressive/anxiolytic medication or a specific treatment by a psychologist, it seems that main ingredients of the rehabilitation program such as physical exercise in many forms and the patient education and support program are the main contributors to the positive change observed among the majority of those patients with symptoms of anxiety and depression.

References

[1] Hemingway, H; Marmot, M. Evidence based cardiology: psychosocial factors in the aetiology and prognosis of coronary heart disease. Systematic review of prospective cohort studies. *BMJ.*, 1999, May 29, 318(7196), 1460-1467.

[2] Frasure-Smith, N; Lesperance, F; Talajic, M. Depression following myocardial infarction. Impact on 6-month survival. *JAMA*, 1993, Oct 20, 270(15), 1819-1825.

[3] Hance, M; Carney, RM; Freedland, KE; Skala, J. Depression in patients with coronary heart disease. A 12-month follow-up. Gen.Hosp. *Psychiatry*, 1996, Jan; 18(1), 61-65.

[4] Kawachi, I; Sparrow, D; Vokonas, PS; Weiss, ST. Symptoms of anxiety and risk of coronary heart disease. The Normative Aging Study. *Circulation*, 1994, Nov, 90(5), 2225-2229.

[5] Rozanski, A; Blumenthal, JA; Kaplan, J. Impact of psychological factors on the pathogenesis of cardiovascular disease and implications for therapy. *Circulation*, 1999, Apr 27; 99(16), 2192-2217.

[6] Zigmond, AS; Snaith, RP. The hospital anxiety and depression scale. Acta Psychiatr. *Scand.*, 1983 Jun; 67(6), 361-370.

[7] Strik, JJ; Honig, A; Lousberg, R; Denollet, J. Sensitivity and specificity of observer and self-report questionnaires in major and minor depression following myocardial infarction. *Psychosomatics*, 2001, Sep-Oct; 42(5), 423-428.

[8] Goldberg, R; Hillberg, R; Reinecker, L; Goldstein, R. Evaluation of patients with severe pulmonary disease before and after pulmonary rehabilitation. Disabil. *Rehabil.*, 2004, Jun 3; 26(11), 641-648.

[9] Benediktsdottir, B; Tomasson, K; Gislason, T. Climateric symptoms and hormone replacement treatment among 50 years old Icelandic women. *Laeknabladid*, 2000, July/August; 86(7/8), 501-507.

[10] Lavie, CJ; Milani, RV. Adverse psychological and coronary risk profiles in young patients with coronary artery disease and benefits of formal cardiac rehabilitation. Arch.Intern.Med. 2006, Sep 25, 166(17), 1878-1883.

[11] Helgason, T; Tomasson, K; Sigfusson, E; Zoega, T. Screening for mental disorders in the community 1984 and 2002 and prescriptions for

psychopharmaca in 1984 and 2001. *Laeknabladid*, 2004 Jul; 90(7/8), 553-559.

[12] Todaro, JF; Shen, BJ; Raffa, SD; Tilkemeier, PL; Niaura, R. Prevalence of anxiety disorders in men and women with established coronary heart disease. J.Cardiopulm.Rehabil. *Prev.*, 2007 Mar-Apr; 27(2), 86-91.

In: Cardiac Rehabilitaiton
Editor: J. T. Halliday, pp. 211-218
ISBN: 978-1-60741-918-1

Chapter X

Cardiac Rehabilitation in Children with Congenital Heart Disease

Tony Reybrouck [*] ***and Marc Gewillig***
Departments of Cardiovascular Rehabilitation and Pediatric Cardiology, Gasthuisberg University Hospital and Department of Rehabilitation Sciences, University of Leuven, KU Leuven, 3000 Leuven, Belgium

Abstract

As the majority of the patients with congenital heart disease belong to the paediatric age group, exercise testing equipment and exercise protocols have to be adapted for children.

Functional performance should be assessed by performing exercise testing with measurement of gas exchange. Nowadays, new concepts for exercise testing in the paediatric age group are analysis of gas exchange during the non-steady state of exercise and determination of the kinetics of gas exchange during the recovery phase of exercise.

* Correspondence: Department of Cardiovascular Rehabilitation Gasthuisberg University Hospital Herestraat 3000 Leuven Belgium, E mail: tony.reybrouck@uz.kuleuven.ac.be, Phone : +32 16 342181, Fax : +32 16 342184

In some groups of patients with congenital heart disease, suboptimal values have been found for aerobic exercise capacity, which can be ascribed to hemodynamic dysfunction or residual hemodynamic lesions after surgery (e.g. in transposition of the great arteries, tetralogy of Fallot, and Fontan repair for univentricular heart). In other types of pathologies medically imposed restriction of intensive physical exercise or competitive sports may determine to some extent a subnormal value of exercise performance.

Finally in some other types of congenital heart disease without overt hemodynamic dysfunction (e.g. ventricular septal defect or atrial septal defect, with normal pressures in the pulmonary circulation) a suboptimal value for aerobic capacity is often related to overprotection of the parents or environment of the child. Therefore, except for some cases with medically imposed restriction of intensive physical exercise, most patients are encouraged to be fully active during leisure time and to participate in all types of physical exercise at school.

Exercise intensity is usually defined as the highest level of physical activity at which the child is still able to talk during physical activity

Formal rehabilitation programs are generally indicated after surgical correction of the defect during the hospitalisation period.

Introduction

Beneficial effects of exercise have been documented in healthy adults and also in adult patients with ischemic heart disease. Also children with congenital heart disease are encouraged to exercise and to be fully active after corrective surgery. These recommendations are based on clinical observations which have shown favourable effects of physical activity in the children and for the parents. In general training effects consist of an increase in the physical working capacity and a more efficient cardiovascular function (lower heart rate response at rest and during exercise), which result in a deceased work of the heart during each systole. Besides these favourable physiological effects, physical rehabilitation in these children has also important psychological advantages. Both patients and parents may be reassured and are not longer afraid from physical activity or exercise. Children and their parents understand that they can participate in normal physical activities, even after a corrective surgical intervention for congenital heart disease.

Exercise Testing in Children with Congenital Heart Disease

Exercise testing in adults has focused mainly on ischemic heart disease. The exercise ECG is helpful in diagnosing the presence or absence of ischemic heart disease [1]. In children the type of pathology is different. The majority of children will present with congenital heart disease.

Exercise testing has shown to be more sensitive in assessing the functional capacity than history taking or questionnaires about physical activity. Usually questionnaires do not evaluate the intensity of exercise and do not give an objective assessment of exercise capacity. A considerable number of patients overestimate their functional performance capacity. When using recall questionnaires to classify the children as active or non-active, both parents and children misclassified themselves in about 30 % of the cases, when correlated with objective measurements of maximal oxygen uptake [2,3]. A larger number of patients show reduced level of daily physical activity. For example in patients who underwent total correction of tetralogy of Fallot and who were clinically well, significantly lower levels of daily physical activity are found, assessed by a questionnaire in boys (Table 1) [4].

Conventional parameters to assess functional capacity in children with congenital heart disease are maximal oxygen uptake or peak oxygen uptake and ventilatory anaerobic threshold.

Table I. Habitual level of physical activity in normal children and in patients 13 girls and 26 boys after surgical repair of tetralogy of Fallot

	Normal children	*Patients*	
Girls	4.26 (3.9-4.8)	2.19 (1-4)	$p < 0.001$
Boys	4.37 (3.3-6.9)	3.74 (1.5-6.5)	$p < 0.05$

The habitual level of physical activity is expressed as a score based on a questionnaire.

* Statistical analysis was performed after logarithmic transformation of the values to normalize the distribution of data. Therefore the geometric mean and the range are reported. Modified from Reybrouck et al [4]

The maximal oxygen uptake gives an objective assessment of the functional reserve capacity of the cardiovascular system and is dependent on maximal cardiac output and arterio-venous oxygen difference. In children with congenital heart disease the maximal cardiac output can be decreased which leads to low values of maximal oxygen uptake e.g. in patients with Fontan operation for univentricular heart, this means a bypass is made from the caval veins to the pulmonary arteries, with no right ventricular pump.

Cardiac Rehabilitation in Children with Congenital Heart Disease

Children with congenital heart disease in whom corrective surgery has been performed, are advised to perform a graded exercise rehabilitation program. In the past the situation was comparable to patients with myocardial infarction. Clinicians thought that it was more prudent for these patients to avoid intensive physical exercise during six weeks, until the lesions of the thoracotomy were healed. After that time children were allowed to resume previous activities. From clinical studies it has been shown that many children who underwent surgical correction of congenital heart disease never became fully active [3,4]. Therefore in recent documents of the European Society of Cardiology, guidelines have been formulated with recommendations and restrictions of physical activity in children and adolescents with congenital heart disease [6,7]. These recommendations are based on clinical findings, which have shown that physical exercise in children with congenital heart defects has beneficial effects on the physical, psychological and socal levels both for the children and for the parents. The risk of physical exercise is low [6].

- In hospital rehabilitation

After surgical correction of a congenital heart defect a formal rehabilitation program is usually performed. This consists of chest physiotherapy (breathing exercises) and early mobilization. The children perform exercises on a cycle ergometer or a treadmill, and can walk in the corridors of the hospital. An easy rule to determine the intensity of exercise is the talk test [8] : this means the patients can perform exercises as long as they still are able to talk during exercise to each other or to the therapist. A soon as the children are discharged from the hospital they are encouraged to resume their previous normal physical activities at home.

- Physical training in children with congenital heart disease

Because children have a natural need to play and like to participate in strenuous activity or competitive sports, some guidelines should be formulated to know whether exercise can be harmful for patients with congenital heart disease.

Clinical studies have shown that children show the same adaptations to training compared to adults [9]. Bar-Or and Rowland reviewed several studies on the effect of physical training on the cardiovascular exercise performance, in children with different types of congenital heart disease such as transposition of the great arteries, tetralogy of Fallot after correction and single ventricle, compared to normal controls. In this analysis they found an average increase in physical working capacity of 21 % compared to 30 % in the normal children. The VO2 max increased by 11 % in children with congenital heart disease. In some studies an increase in maximal working capacity was found without an increase in VO2 max. [10,11]. This has been attributed to the fact that the efficiency of the oxygen uptake could be improved which leads to a higher physical performance for a same level of oxygen uptake. It could be that irreversible damage of the cardiovascular system has occurred, which leads to an inability to increase the maximal oxygen uptake.

An important observation for exercise rehabilitation studies in children with congenital heart disease is the high dropout rate. Therefore children and also parents need to be motivated to continue this exercise training programs. To improve compliance to the exercise program several rules can be followed:

- Exercise sessions should be performed at the same time of the day
- The child should be accompanied by a family member during exercise training
- For exercise programs it is important that the children have a warming up period and after exercise a cool down period at lower exercise intensity to prevent presyncope after exercise

- Exercise intensity should not be too excessive in order to avoid demotivation of the child. A useful tool is the talk test: the children should still be able to talk during exercise.

B. Specific Guidelines for Exercise and Sports Participation in Children with Congenital Heart Disease

Every patient, parent of physician should know what the patient can and may do.

- In some pathologies the patient can and may do everything as his peers, e.g. postoperative closure of an atrial septal defect or a ventricular septal defect, closed ducts, mild pulmonary stenosis. In these cases no restrictions have to be recommended.
- Problems can arise if a patient can do more than he may do, when he exceeds the limits of safe activity e.g. aortic stenosis, postoperative Fallot, Senning operation for transposition of the great arteries, Fontan operation (RAPA), coarctation of the aorta, coronary abnormalities, pulmonary hypertension.
- Less problematic are patients who can do little effort and therefore may do exercise as they can as they are "auto-limited", e.g. Fontan operation (TCPC), Eisenmenger syndrome, palliated cyanotic heart disease.

Conclusion

Children with successful repair of congenital heart disease are frequently less active than healthy peers. Some children may complain of early onset of fatigue during physical exercise, which may be related to some degree of deconditioning in many cases. Only a minority has a medical imposed restriction of physical activity. Therefore these children and parents should be encouraged to participate in physical exercise programs. Because it is difficult to formulate general guidelines, these recommendations are intended to support the clinician to offer advice in making clinical decisions.

References

[1] Gibbons, RJ; Balady, GJ; Beasley, JW; Bricker, JT; Duvernoy, WFC; Froelichter, VF; et al. ACC/AHA Guidelines for Exercise Testing. A Report of the American College of Cardiology/American Heart Association Task force on Practice Guidelines (Committee on Exercise Testing). *J Am Coll Cardiol,* 1997, 30, 260-315.

[2] Rogers, R; Reybrouck, T; Weymans, M; Dumoulin, M; Van der Hauwaert L, Gewillig M. Reliability of subjective estimates of exercise capacity after total repair of tetralogy of Fallot. *Acta Paediatr,* 1994, 83, 866-9.

[3] Barber, G; Heise, CT. Subjective estimates of exercise ability: Comparison to objective measurements. *Pediatr Exerc Sci* 1991, 3, 327-32.

[4] Reybrouck, T; Weymans, M; Stijns, H; van der Hauwaert, LG. Exercise testing after correction of tetralogy of Fallot: The fallacy of a reduced heart rate response. *Am Heart J,* 1986, 112, 998-1003.

[5] Reybrouck, T; Roger, R; Weymans, M; Dumoulin, M; Vanhove, M; Daenen, W; et al. Serial exercise testing in patients with congenital heart disease. *Eur J Pediatr,* 1995, 154, 801-6.

[6] Hirth, A; Reybrouck, T; Bjarnason-Wehrens, B; Lawrenz, W; Hoffmann, A. Recommendations for participation in competitive and leisure sports in patients with congenital heart disease. *Eur J Cardiovasc Prevent Rehab,* 2006, 13, 293-299.

[7] Pelliccia, A; Fagard, R; BjØrnstad, HH; Anastassakis, A; Arbustini, E; Assanelli, D; et al. Recommendations for competitive sports participation in athletes with cardiovascular disease : a consensus document from the Study Group of Sports Cardiology of the Working Group of Cardiac Rehabilitation and Exercise Physiology and the Working Group of Myocardial and Pericardial Diseases of the European Society of Cardiology. *Eur Heart J,* 2005, 26(14), 1422-45.

[8] Reybrouck, T; Mertens, L. Physical performance and physical activity in grown-up congenital heart disease. *Eur J Cardiov Prevent Rehab,* 2005, 12, 498-502.

[9] Bar-Or, O; Rowland, TW. Physiologic and perceptual responses to exercise in the healthy child. Pediatric Medicine: From physiologic

principles to health care application. Champaign, IL: Human Kinetics, 2004, p. 3-61,

[10] Balfour, IC; Drimma, AM; Nouri, S; Pennington, DG; Hemkens, C; Harvey, LL. Pediatric cardiac rehabilitation. *A J D C,* 1991, 145, 627-630.

[11] Ruttenberg, H; Moller, JH; Strong, WB; Fisher, AG; Adams, TD. Recommended guidelines for graded exercise testing and exercise presentation in children with heart disease. *J Cardiac Rehab,* 1984, 4, 10-16.

Index

A

B

C

E

F

G

H

I

J

K

L

M

N

O

P

Q

R

S

T